# The Facts About Fats

# The FACTS ABOUT FATS

## A Consumer's Guide to Good Oils

JOHN FINNEGAN

CELESTIAL ARTS
BERKELEY, CALIFORNIA

**Reader Please Note:** This material has been written and published solely for educational purposes. It should not be used as a substitute for a physician's advice.

Those who need medical attention are strongly recommended to seek out a physician or practitioner knowledgeable in this field and work under his / her direction.

The author provides this information with the understanding that people act on it at their own risk and with full knowledge that they should consult with health professionals for any help they need.

Text and cover design by Ken Scott
Typesetting by Star Type

FIRST CELESTIAL ARTS PRINTING 1993

Library of Congress Cataloging-in-Publication Data
Finnegan, John.
    The Facts About Fats: a consumer's guide to good oils / John Finnegan.
      p.  cm.
    Includes bibliographical references and index.
    ISBN 0-89087-680-0
    1.  Essential fatty acids in human nutrition.   2.  Fats and oils, Edible.
    3.  Fatty acids in human nutrition.   I.  Title.
QP752.E84F56    1993
612.3'97—dc20
                                                  92-35402
                                                      CIP

3   4   5   6   7   8 / 99   98   97   96   95   94

# Acknowledgments

In this day and age of seemingly endless corruption in our society, it is truly refreshing to find people who have a genuine love and appreciation for life and who care about this earth and the creatures and plants living upon it.

I want to thank the many people who have given so warmly and freely of their time and help in producing this book. I especially want to thank my brother Todd, for his enduring faith and support; to Kathy Cituk, who wrote some of the material and helped edit the text; to Sherry Weinstein ("Slash") whose brilliant editing was essential in bringing this book to completion; Bob Walberg, who has been a continual source of good humor, information, and honesty; Dr. Anine Lorenzen, who drove me all over Europe and who tolerated my eccentric behavior; and Dr. Barbara Bieber, who visited Dr. Budwig with me, spoke with the Kousmine Foundation, and translated their information and replies to my questions, all of which contributed greatly to the comprehensive information contained within this book.

I also want to express my deep thanks to David Hinds, my publisher at Celestial Arts; to Jorgen Uhrskov for his genuine friendship and support; to Dr. Brian Roettger D.C.; and to Thomas Greither, Dr. Michael Winther, Mark Weideman, Dr. Dan Roehm, Dr. Stephen Langer, Seigfreid Gursche, Udo Erasmus, Bill Vincent, Lucia Oswald, Robert Gaffney, Geri Whidden, Mrs. Rudin, Charlotte Gerson, John Hunt, Danielle Fitzpatrick, Linda Reyes, Marlyese Ruess, Francoise Paradis, Willow Parks, Yvon Tremblay, Judy Stepps, Carola Eastwood, Sarah Brennan, Jeffrey Selkov, Jan Buchalter, Dhayanna Gagne, Debra Pearlstein, Dr. Mark Swanson, Gerry Greenberg, John Baier, Stuart Wigderson, and Fred Rohe for his excellent piece on "The Great Margarine Experiment," as well as my many other friends and colleagues who assisted in bringing this book to fruition.

And especially thanks to the Grace.

John Finnegan

# Contents

೨

# Introduction

Over the past 40 years I have seen a marked change in medical opinion of nutrition and the use of nutrients as supplements. In 1950 when I first began to practice medicine, it was generally believed that nutrition played a very minor, if any, role in the practice of medicine. Nutrition was not taught in medical schools, and physicians allowed non-clinical nutritionists and dietitians to take over the entire field.

In 1955 the first paper was published which introduced the concept that large doses of vitamins could be used therapeutically for treating conditions not known to be vitamin deficiency diseases. The decade 1970 to 1980 marked the beginning of the megavitamin decade. The following decade saw the introduction of mineral supplements on a larger scale.

The last decade is properly the essential fatty acid decade. There has been an enormous rise of interest in these fats and oils, and the roles they play in a large number of diseases. This includes the study of cardiovascular disease, the connection to cholesterol and other fats, and most important, the connection to the essential fatty acids.

For this reason this book by John Finnegan is very timely. If we are to use these essential nutrients with skill and safety, it is important that we understand their chemistry, what they do, how they are made, and some of the conditions for which there is clear evidence of their usefulness. It is especially important to know how these oils are made. They are very unstable, i.e. they have double bonds in them which are avid for oxygen. This is why linseed oil is used to make a base for paint. For the same reason, once the oils have been extracted they will not store very well. During their deterioration or oxidation the oils are changed to products which are of no value and which may be harmful. Manufacturers have tried to avoid some of these changes by using what is called a "cold" pressing process, which is supposed to avoid the use of heat. Heat increases oxidation and deterioration. But even when the oil is cold pressed, there is a lot of heat generated in the process unless the oil is pressed so slowly that the heat has a chance to dissipate. This means that the cold pressed oils are little better than the heat treated oils. However there are a few manufacturers who have produced products that are very little deteriorated, and they store their oils under nitrogen until the bottle is opened. All these topics and more are discussed in this important volume.

I recommend this book because it is accurate, factual, easy to read and very informative. With the information available in this book it should be much easier for people to become healthier and to live longer, fuller, and better quality lives.

A. Hoffer, M.D., Ph.D.

# CHAPTER 1

# Our Need for Essential Fatty Acids

## Modern Health and Disease

Today we are witnessing an unprecedented rise of diseases that have never before existed. The health of civilized nations is deteriorating at an accelerated rate. Much has been accomplished in the reduction and control of infectious diseases during this century, due to improved sanitation and housing conditions in our cities, the development and widespread use of antibiotics, and other advances. But we are also witnessing the creation and dramatic increase of degenerative diseases such as heart disease, cancer, arthritis, Candida, diabetes, immune system breakdown, and mental illness, all of which involve a weakening of the normal health, strength, and balance of the organism. Most diseases we face today in Western nations are not those caused by an extremely virulent pathogenic organism like malaria, but rather by a disturbance in homeostasis; a breakdown in integrity, a malfunction in the normal biochemical processes of the body.

Until the early 1900s, illnesses like scurvy (caused by a deficiency of vitamin C), beriberi, and pellagra (caused by deficiencies of vitamin $B^1$ and $B^3$, respectively) were treated by an unknowing medical profession with various therapies, including leeches and electroshock therapy. Today of course, these diseases are successfully treated using vitamin therapy and a good diet.

There is a substantial and growing body of excellent medical and scientific evidence showing that many common diseases (i.e. heart disease, cancer, immune system weakness and depression) are, to a large extent, caused and can be treated by nutrition. Just as, a century ago, scurvy, beriberi, and pellagra existed because of nutritional deficiencies, so also many present-day diseases are partially caused by deficiencies. Heart disease and cancer, our two most common illnesses, account for a million deaths annually in the U.S., as well as leaving millions of others disabled, at a cost of billions of dollars. These illnesses arise largely from nutritional deficiencies, especially of the Omega-3 fatty acids, compounded by damage from poisons in our foods and environment (especially the toxic trans fatty acids and free radicals in refined oils). But these and other illnesses are now being successfully treated with nutrition, herbs, and other therapies, and hopefully will be treatable, if not preventable, in the future.

One hundred years ago, heart disease was virtually non-existent. The first recorded case of coronary occlusion appeared in medical literature in 1910. Today, two-thirds of the population in the U.S. develops heart disease. One hundred years ago, Alzheimer's disease was nonexistent. Today, it is the fourth leading cause of death. One hundred years ago, cancer caused only 3.4 percent of all deaths in Europe and the U.S. Today, one in three people get cancer (up from one in ten a decade ago), and one in four die from it. A century ago, only one person in one hundred thousand in the U.S. had diabetes; today one in twenty have it.[1]

These are powerful statistics, a strong message to us that something has gone very wrong with the way we are living.

It is critical that we live with more respect and appreciation for the gift of our creation and the basic laws, values, and harmony of nature; that we stop abusing our world and ignoring the precious, fragile nutrients created by life along the food chain.

# Our Need for Essential Fatty Acids

There is a widespread realization that our foods and our diets have become seriously deficient in key minerals, vitamins, fiber, amino acids, and often complex carbohydrates. Yet only now is it becoming generally understood that modern processing methods of fats and oils have created even more serious damage from poisonous, rancid oils and trans fatty acids, as well as deficiencies of Omega-3 and Omega-6 fatty acids and certain prostaglandins.

The key to understanding the fats, oils, and cholesterol controversy is balance. The body is made from, and requires, cholesterol and the Omega-3 and Omega-6 fatty acids. It needs an entire range of minerals, proteins, and vitamins. When there is too much or too little of any of these ingredients, disorder and disease will result.

Just as we need good quality proteins, carbohydrates, vitamins, and minerals, we also need good quality fats and oils for physical and mental health. There are two types of fats, saturated and unsaturated. The saturated fats, found in butter, eggs, fish, chicken, and meats, are generally high in cholesterol. The unsaturated fats are found in vegetable oils, such as sunflower, sesame, safflower, corn, and flax seed oil. These are high in the essential Omega-6 and Omega-3 fatty acids. The nonessential monosaturated fatty acids are found in olive and other oils.

We need a certain amount of both saturated and unsaturated fats in our diets. Except for people who have advanced heart disease from a lifetime of poor eating and little exercise, most of us need a minimal amount of cholesterol in our diet. Over 8 percent of our brain's solid matter is made of cholesterol. Our hormones, skin, and even the membranes of our cells use cholesterol as an essential building block in their basic production and structure.[2,3,4,5,6]

We also need the unsaturated fats—Omega-6 and Omega-3 fatty acids found in the vegetable oils. It isn't a question of either/or—should I use saturated or unsaturated fats? Most of us need both in good quality forms. What we don't need are the refined or hydrogenated fats found in margarines, vegetable shortenings, and refined vegetable oils.

People who previously had excellent health when living on a traditional diet of unprocessed foods, begin to succumb to the plethora of degenerative diseases of modern civilization after moving to a civilized nation and adopting the eating and living habits of their peers. Ewan Cameron, Director of the Cancer Nutriprevention Project at the Linus Pauling Institute of Science and Medicine, wrote,

> Heart disease and cancer are the leading causes of death in the United States and Europe. Both heart disease and cancer have been separately linked on a country-by-country basis to the amount of fat consumed.
>
> But there are some puzzling exceptions. Japanese women consuming traditional Japanese diets have only a quarter of the breast cancer incidence of United States women, but the daughters of Japanese immigrants to the U.S., acquiring Western dietary habits, soon have the same breast cancer incidence as their new compatriots, hence, ruling out genetic factors. Also, both heart disease and cancer are practically unknown among Greenland Eskimos who, in the native state, have probably the highest per capita fat consumption in the world. However, the fat in both traditional Japanese and Eskimo diets comes mainly from marine rather than terrestrial (seed oils and animal fats) sources. I wondered about a common dietary factor between heart disease and cancer.[7]

He then carried out the same double-blind study twice on cancer-prone mice. The mice that were fed flax seed oil (containing Omega-3 and Omega-6) developed almost no tumors. The other mice were fed oils that were refined and did not have a balance of both these fats, including GLA (gamma linolenic acid), and were found to have enhanced tumor growth. This study shows both the importance of having a balance of Omega-3 and Omega-6 fats in our diets, and using unrefined oils in the prevention and treatment of cancer.

In recent years, Dr. Catherine Kousmine, Dr. Johanna Budwig, Udo Erasmus, Dr. Donald Rudin, Ann Louise Gittleman, and others have shown the critical need for the Omega-6 and Omega-3 fatty acids in our diets. These fats are good sources of energy. They are an essential part of the body's oxygen transport mechanism as well as being key building blocks of our cells and hormones. They also play a vital role in many other key body structures and processes.

Most of us obtain ample (and often excessive) amounts of the Omega-6 fatty acids from safflower, sesame, sunflower, soy, canola, and corn oils, but are deficient in the Omega-3 fatty acids. The only true concentrated sources of the Omega-3 fatty acids are flax seed oil; certain fish, such as mackerel, sardines, tuna, trout, and cold water salmon; and to a lesser degree, unrefined canola and walnut oils. A deficiency of Omega-3s has been strongly implicated as a main cause of heart disease, cancer, immune system breakdown and other modern maladies. These fats must be present in our diet to maintain good health.

1. Joseph D. Weissman, M.D., "The X Factor," *New Age Journal* (March / April 1988): 42.
2. Ann Louise Gittleman, M.A., *Beyond Pritikin* (New York: Bantam, 1989).
3. Rudolph Ballentine, M.D., "Butter vs. Oil," *East / West Journal* (February 1988).
4. Bruce Alberts, et al., *Molecular Biology of the Cell* (New York: Garland Publishing, Inc., 1989).
5. Robert B. Gennis, *Biomembranes Molecular Structure and Function* (New York: Springer-Verlag, 1989).
6. Charles Bates, Ph.D., *Essential Fatty Acids and Immunity in Mental Health* (Washington: Life Sciences Press, 1987).
7. Ewan Cameron, Director, Cancer Nutriprevention Project, Linus Pauling Institute of Science and Medicine, (June 10, 1987). (A study.)

# CHAPTER 2

# Causes of Essential Fatty Acid Deficiency

T he dramatic changes in dietary habits and in agricultural, food processing, and food preparation methods that have occurred over the past one hundred years have brought about an unprecedented alteration in our nourishment. This has had serious consequences, creating a vast increase in degenerative illnesses in nearly all technologically developed societies.

Following are the major changes that have caused the deficiency of essential fatty acids (EFAs) today:

**1. Change in flour milling technology,** causing rancidity and elimination of essential fatty acids.

**2. Elimination of Omega-3 foods, such as flax seed oil, because of limited shelf life.** Marketers have eliminated flax seed oil and other oils with a high content of Omega-3 fats because of their limited shelf life with their bottling methods.

**3. Change to feedlot-raised cattle as a primary protein source along with caged chickens and their eggs.** Change from wild game, free-range cattle, deer, turkey, sheep, fish, etc., to cage-raised cattle, chicken, their eggs, and dairy products as main protein sources. Free-range cattle, chicken, their eggs, and dairy products can have up to five times as much Omega-3 and Omega-6 fats in their tissues, and a much lower amount of hard cholesterol fats than their caged counterparts.[1]

The same change has happened to farm-raised rainbow trout, shrimp, and salmon, all of which normally have a high content of EFAs and their derivatives. When grown on fish farms, their EFA content is substantially reduced. This is because their normal foods—small fish such as minnows, krill (tiny shrimp), algae, insects, and insect larvae, all high in EFAs—are replaced with grain-based meals and other less nutritious foods.

**4. Certain groups of people have an inherited need for more EFAs and GLA (gamma linolenic acid) in their diet.** The genetic heritage of these population groups—Celtic Irish, Scottish, Welsh, Scandinavian, Danish, British Columbian coastal Indians, and Eskimos—predisposes them to need more EFAs in their diets. This is because their ancestors lived on large amounts of fish, high in these nutrients. They are much more prone to develop deficiency diseases when their diets lack sufficient quantities of these key nutrients.[2, 3]

**5. Increased use of drugs and pharmaceuticals,** particularly aspirin, that block EFA enzyme systems and their conversion to vital prostaglandins.

**6. Increased use of sugar, caffeine, refined carbohydrates, and alcohol,** which deplete EFAs and prostaglandins. Alcohol and caffeine also block conversion of EFAs to prostaglandins.

**7. Increased ingestion of toxins in food, water, and air,** which deplete EFAs.

**8. Lack of breast feeding.** Omega-3 fats and DHA (docosahexaenoic acid) are not present in infant formulas or commercial cow's milk. They are deficient, also, in the breast-milk of mothers whose diets are deficient in Omega-3 fatty acids.

**9. Excessive consumption of Omega-6 fatty acids,** which interferes with the absorption of Omega-3 fatty acids.

**10. Excessive consumption of trans fatty acids and hydrogenated fats.** Marketers want products that last for months, if not years, on the supermarket shelf. They have introduced refined and hydrogenated oils, which are high in poisonous trans fatty acids, rancid fats, and free radicals, and deficient in vital Omega-3 and Omega-6 fatty acids. The average Western person today consumes 1000 percent more trans fatty acids and hydrogenated fats than ever before.[4]

෨

1.  Donald O. Rudin, M.D., *The Omega-3 Phenomenon* (New York: Rawson Associates, 1987).
2.  Ibid.
3.  Charles Bates, Ph.D., *Essential Fatty Acids and Immunity in Mental Health* (Washington: Life Sciences Press, 1987).
4.  Rudin, op. cit.

CHAPTER 3

# The Revolution in Oil Production

## The History of Oil Production

For hundreds of years, until the 1900s, cultures around the world have utilized simple and effective means of extracting oils from seeds, nuts, and fruits. In Europe, every village had at least one oil beater. The oil beater would put flax or other seeds into a funnel, place a steel wedge on top of the seeds, and then pound the wedge with a sledge hammer—crushing the seeds and pressing the oil into a container. Then, once or twice a week, he would put the barrel of oil onto his wagon and drive his horse through the village streets selling fresh-pressed oil door-to-door, just as other farmers would bring fresh milk, eggs, and vegetables.

Oil was considered a perishable product to be utilized soon after pressing. In the home it was often stored in ceramic containers which allowed no light to enter, and was kept in a cool, dark place.

The difference in the basic consciousness towards food in America and most European countries is striking. In Europe, bread can only be sold as "fresh" on the day that it is made. After that, it is sold as "day-old bread" for one day only, and then must be discarded. In America, bread labeled "fresh" often sits on the supermarket shelves for a week.

Most of the oils made in Europe, while not nearly as well made as they once were, are still less refined and of a far superior quality than the commercial oils made in the U.S. Olive oil was traditionally made (and still is for the extra virgin oil) by simple pressing methods. The process was held in the highest regard by the peoples of the Mediterranean countries.

In Asia, they developed a method of extracting oils by building a large wooden mortar and pestle with a hole in the bottom. They would fill the bowl of the pestle with seed (flax, mustard, and others). Then, they would hitch an ox, camel, or water buffalo to the end of a long pole attached to the mortar, and walk him in circles around the pestle, crushing the seeds and allowing the oil to drip through into a container placed below. In Southeast Asia, oil was extracted from the palm fruit by simply boiling it in large pots of water, and then skimming off the oil after it had cooled.

Some tribes of American Indians developed a simple method to extract the oil from seeds by putting the seeds into a wooden funnel, placing a rock on top of the seeds, and then hammering the rock with another rock until the seeds were crushed and the oil dripped into the waiting bowl below.

For centuries, people have enjoyed oils extracted by very simple methods that didn't create toxic by-products. Oil was treated as a highly perishable food, used quickly after pressing and stored in light-insulated containers, usually ceramic.

Then came the industrial revolution. Huge machines and chemical processes were created so that oils could be mass-produced in clear glass and plastic containers, to sit on shelves for months on end without going rancid.

## Refined Oils: The Industrial Revolution

How did industrial engineers accomplish this feat of making "food" that won't age or go bad? It was easy—they developed very sophisticated chemical refining processes that removed or destroyed nearly all life-sustaining nutrients present in oils so they could sit almost indefinitely without decaying. But, these clever refining methods also created many poisonous compounds like trans fatty acids, free radicals, and other toxic substances.

And today we have, wonder of wonders, margarine—"the perfect spread"—a food that can sit on your windowsill for years, exposed to the elements and infectious agents of nature and not show a whit of decay; something that no mold or yeast will grow on, no insect will lay its eggs in, no rodent will touch; something that not even the cockroaches will eat.

A front page article in the October 1992 New York Times cited new studies which have found that margarine and vegetable shortening, and other products made from partially hydrogenated vegetable oils made from soybean and corn may cause heart disease.[1]

While one of the biggest fallacies is that margarines and other refined vegetable oils are good for our hearts and health, even more deceptive is the false representation by major health food oil producers that they supply pure, unheated, nutritious cooking and salad oils.

For years, even decades, I have gone into health food stores and bought my sesame, safflower, and other oils, assured that I was purchasing good quality, health-promoting foods for cooking and salad dressings. Imagine my shock when I discovered that the public has been sold a bill of goods regarding the purity, safety, and nutritional value of these so-called "health food" oils. This situation is similar to one that occurred some years ago. There was a health food mayonnaise that everyone raved about and thought was a delicious, high quality health food product until one day a newspaper article revealed that the government had closed the plant because it was discovered that they had taken regular, brand name commercial mayonnaise, removed the labels, put on their own health food labels, and then sold it to an unknowing public.

The same situation exists now with many health food oils. Most companies do not make their own oils. They buy them from the same giant corporations that produce the commercial oils (made by nearly the same methods), bottle them and put on health food labels which read "cold-processed" and then sell them at inflated prices. The problem is, that while they advertise these oils as being cold-processed from an expeller press (which means pressed at temperatures of 140–160 degrees F and higher), these oils are actually refined (at temperatures up to 500 degrees F). This creates poisonous fats and free radicals, and seriously damages the vital nutrients in the oils.

Refined oils are subjected to several processing methods: deodorization, winterizing, bleaching, and alkali refining.[2,3,4,5] These processes remove virtually all of the vitamin E, lecithin, and beta carotene from the oil. Worse yet, refining destroys much of the Omega-3 and Omega-6 essential fatty acids, converting them into poisonous trans fatty acids.[6,7,8] Many studies have shown how trans fatty acids are a major cause of heart disease and cancer.[9,10] Dr. Donald Rudin, Ann Louse Gittleman, and other researchers have also shown the poisonous effects of trans fats, as well as a recent study conducted in the Netherlands by two Dutch scientists, published in the *New England Journal of Medicine*.[11]

Their research revealed that trans fatty acids (from refined oils) increase the LDL (or bad) cholesterol as much as saturated fats do and they lower the HDL (or good) cholesterol. Even the saturated fats do not reduce the HDL cholesterol.[12] This study confirms what many people have thought. If anything contributes to heart disease and cancer, it is these plasticized foods— margarine and refined cooking and salad oils. According to the *New York Times* article,

> Industry officials and the Federal Government contend that Americans eat far fewer trans fatty acids—no more than 8 to 10 grams a day—than the participants in the Dutch study, who consumed 34 grams. In the Agriculture Department

study the participants consumed 8 to 20 grams of trans fatty acids.

Dr. Mary Enig, a former research associate in the department of chemistry and biochemistry at the University of Maryland and now a nutrition consultant in Silver Spring, Md. says the industry figure is low.

Dr. Enig, who has studied trans fatty acids for decades, analyzed more than 600 foods to determine their trans fatty acid content. Americans eat 11 to 28 grams of trans fatty acids a day, she said, which is as much as 20 percent of the fat they eat daily.

Dr. Enig found 8 grams of trans fatty acids in a large order of french fries cooked in partially hydrogenated vegetable oil, 10 grams in a typical serving of fast-food, fried chicken, or fried fish, and eight grams in two ounces of imitation cheese.[13]

Refined oils also develop a certain amount of rancidity because they are processed in the presence of light and oxygen. Then they are bottled in clear glass containers, which allow the light to penetrate and further their rancidity.[14,15] Light causes serious free radical damage to oils, and light oxidation is much faster than oxygen oxidation.[16]

The deodorizing phase of the refining process is the worst. The oil is subjected to steam distillation at temperatures as high as 470–518 degrees F, which removes the taste of the seed from the oil.[17,18] Why do these companies advertise that their oils are extracted at a low temperature? (Even 140–160 degrees F is high enough to cause some damage to the oils; ideally, they should be produced at temperatures below 118 degrees F.) Why is it necessary to deodorize the oils anyway? I like the taste of the seeds from which they are obtained. Many oils used in Australia, and many oils used in Europe are unrefined.

## Fresh-pressed Organic Oils:
## A Revolution in Oil Production

In 1987, things began to change. Almost simultaneously, two groups in Vancouver, B.C. began researching and developing the technology to produce and bottle good quality vegetable oils from certified organic seeds. Omega Nutrition and Flora, Inc. each spent months of hard work, and trial and error, reworking small oil presses in order to produce a good quality, organic flax seed oil. Much research and innovation was necessary to develop what was to become the first large-scale production of a full line of properly made and bottled, certified organic vegetable oils. In 1990, I was privileged to visit both companies and tour their U.S. and Canadian oil production facilities. I saw firsthand how the oils are produced, and learned the history of each of the different innovations essential to making these oils available.

A new method was invented to press the seeds so the oil is not exposed to either light or oxygen as it flows from the crushed seed into light-excluding containers, and then is sealed with an inert gas so it can be stored properly without going rancid.

Presses were redesigned so the pressing temperatures never exceed 118 degrees F. Gaskets were created out of special materials that will not break down from constant friction and contaminate the oils. A safe material was found in which to bottle the oils without allowing in light.

Farmers were found who would grow the seeds by organic methods. Guarantees were given to buy their crops each year so they could safely convert or continue in organic growing methods.

Distributors and stores were contacted and informed of this vital new understanding, and about an essential nutrient missing from refined oils. And finally, a wary and confused public was presented with clear new information about this exciting development in oil production.

There is one company in Australia that produces oils properly and ships them to Europe. Two companies in Canada and the United States produce oils that meet these standards of quality: Flora, Inc.; and Omega Nutrition. Flora distributes truly fresh-pressed, cold-processed, unrefined oils and packages them in dark glass bottles (a great improvement). However, there is substantial evidence that damaging light rays do penetrate the dark amber glass, causing a certain amount of rancidity.[19,20,21,22] Metal does not make a good container for oil either, because it contaminates the oil. The best solution is to package it in either black glass or a special black plastic container that keeps all light out, and is proven to allow no transmigration of hydrocarbons into the oil.[23,24,25]

Arrowhead Mills distributes the full line of Omega Nutrition oils in the United States. The Omega Nutrition / Arrowhead Mills oils have the added advantage of being the only oils bottled in completely light-excluding containers, and are the only companies producing a full line of organic, fresh-pressed vegetable oils that have both FVO and OCIA (Farm Verified Organic and Organic Crop Improvement Association) certification. This is a crucial concern today because many companies are falsely representing their products as organic when, in reality, they are not. Without independent third-party certification from a reputable company, consumers have no guarantee of the quality of products they purchase.[26]

The word is getting out about what may be the most important development in natural foods' production since the discovery and production of vitamins. Companies like Natures Symphony and Organic Marketing are producing massage oils and beginning to make lotions for skin care that use the Omega Nutrition oils in their formulas.

Let's hope that as we move from the Industrial Age into the Age of Information, the tides will turn again, and as more and more people have access to more and more information, they will demand that foods be fresh and wholesome. As people become familiar with real oils, they may grow tired of eating oils that are refined and devitalized, and start wanting something fresh, good-tasting, and healthy.

꿍

1. "Now What? U.S. Study Says Margarine May Be Harmful," *New York Times* (October 7, 1992): 1.
2. Donald O. Rudin, M.D., and Clara Felix *The Omega-3 Phenomenon* (New York: Rawson Associates, 1987).
3. Daniel Swern, Editor, *Bailey's Industrial Oil and Fat Products* (New York: John Wiley and Sons, 1979).
4. Ann Louise Gittleman, M.S., *Beyond Pritikin* (New York: Bantam, 1989).
5. Rudin, op. cit.
6. Gunstone, Harwood, and Padly, *The Lipid Handbook* (London: Chapman and Hall, 1986).
7. Gittleman, op. cit.
8. Gunstone, et al., op. cit.
9. Swern, op. cit.
10. Gunstone, et al., op. cit.
11. Mensink and Katan, "Trans Fatty Acids and Lipoprotein Levels," *New England Journal of Medicine,* Vol. 323, No. 7 (Aug. 16, 1990).
12. J.A.F. Faria, U. de Vicosa, and M.K. Mukai, "Use of a Gas Chromatographic Reactor to Study Lipid Photo-oxidation," *J.A.O.C.S.* Vol. 60, No. 1, (1983), Rutgers U., New Jersey.
13. New York Times, op. cit.
14. Pete Vincent, Engineering Researcher/Physicist, Study done at T.R.I.U.M.F. at the University of British Columbia facilities (1987).
15. Y. Yamamoto, E. Niki, R. Tanimura, Y. Kamiya, "Study of Oxidation by Chemiluminescence. IV. Detection of Levels of Lipid Hydroperoxides by Chemiluminescence," *Journal of American Oil Chemists Society,* Vol. 62 (Aug. 1985), Dept. Reac. Chem. Fac. Engr., U. of Tokyo, Japan.
16. K. Warner, T.L. Mounts, "Flavor and Oxidative Stability of Hydrogenated and Unhydrogenated Soybean Oils. Efficacy of Plastic Packaging," *Journal of American Oil Chemists Society,* Vol. 61 (Mar. 1984), N.R.R.C., Agr. Research Ser., USDA.
17. Independent testing done by Cantest, Vancouver, B.C., showing no transmigration of hydrocarbons from black plastic containers used by Omega Nutrition.
18. Gittleman, op. cit.
19. Rudolph Ballentine, M.D., "Butter vs. Oil," *East/West Journal* (February 1988).
20. Claudio Galli, and Artemis P. Simopoulos, *Dietary Omega-3 and Omega-6 Fatty Acids: Biological Effects and Nutritional Essentiality* (New York and London: Plenum Press, 1988).
21. Faria, et al., op. cit.
22. Vincent, op. cit.
23. Yamamoto, et al., op. cit.
24. Warner, et al., op. cit.
25. Independent testing done by Cantest, Vancouver, B.C., op. cit.
26. Theodore Wood Carlat, *Organically Grown Food* (California: Wood Publishing, 1990).

# How Oils Are Manufactured

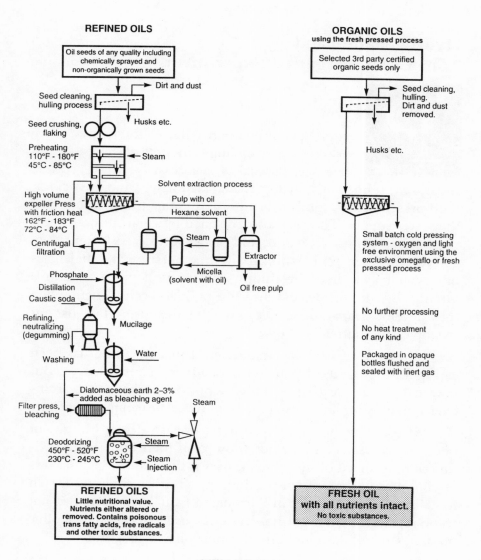

**REFINED OILS**

Oil seeds of any quality including chemically sprayed and non-organically grown seeds

→ Dirt and dust

Seed cleaning, hulling process

Seed crushing, flaking — Husks etc.

Preheating 110°F - 180°F 45°C - 85°C ← Steam

High volume expeller Press with friction heat 162°F - 183°F 72°C - 84°C

Solvent extraction process

Pulp with oil

Hexane solvent

Centrifugal filtration

Steam

Extractor

Micella (solvent with oil)

Oil free pulp

Phosphate
Distillation
Caustic soda

Refining, neutralizing (degumming) — Mucilage

Washing — Water

Diatomaceous earth 2–3% added as bleaching agent

Steam

Filter press, bleaching

Deodorizing 450°F - 520°F 230°C - 245°C — Steam
— Steam Injection

**REFINED OILS**
Little nutritional value.
Nutrients either altered or removed. Contains poisonous trans fatty acids, free radicals and other toxic substances.

**ORGANIC OILS**
using the fresh pressed process

Selected 3rd party certified organic seeds only

→ Seed cleaning, hulling. Dirt and dust removed.

Husks etc.

Small batch cold pressing system - oxygen and light free environment using the exclusive omegaflo or fresh pressed process

No further processing

No heat treatment of any kind

Packaged in opaque bottles flushed and sealed with inert gas

**FRESH OIL**
**with all nutrients intact.**
No toxic substances.

© 1993 John Finnegan

CHAPTER 5

# Butter vs. Margarine

## Hydrogenation and
## "The Great Margarine Experiment"

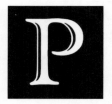

People spend their entire lives—forty, fifty, sixty years—ingesting huge amounts of steaks, french fries, milk shakes, processed cheese, coffee, sugar, salt, refined oils, hydrogenated fats, margarine, pesticides, food preservatives, food colorings, and chlorine and fluoride in the water supply. They are also poisoned by cigarettes, alcohol, recreational drugs, radiation, and pharmaceuticals. Often, they get very little exercise and have lifetime nutritional deficiencies of key nutrients like chromium, magnesium, zinc, selenium, vitamin E, vitamin B6, and the Omega-3 fatty acid. Then, when they develop heart disease, they say, "It's the butter. I've just got to stop eating butter."

Butter is a good wholesome food that mankind has been eating for thousands of years without adverse consequences. But now, people eat margarine—a lifeless poison, packed with carcinogens, fit only for lubricating the front wheel bearings of your car.

If someone has developed heart disease after a lifetime of poor eating habits and malnutrition, or if their body has a malfunctioning metabolism which causes it to create large amounts of cholesterol, then of course, butter and other cholesterol-rich foods should be reduced or eliminated from their diet. But not to be replaced by margarine. Better to use a good quality olive oil, flax seed oil, hazelnut oil, or canola oil as a substitute.

The best story I have ever heard that gives a sense of the

margarine fiasco is called **"The Great Margarine Experiment,"** done by Fred Rohe. Fred Rohe is a well-known figure in the natural foods movement, and is the author of *The Zen of Running, Dr. Kelley's Answer to Cancer,* and *The Complete Book of Natural Foods.* Living in a remote area of northern California, he operates an advertising agency called Organic Marketing, and is a marketing consultant to the natural foods industry. Following is the historic study in his own words.

## The Great Margarine Experiment

"Between 1965 and 1973, I owned a couple of natural foods stores, one in San Francisco, California, and one in Palo Alto. One day, I was talking to a food technologist who shopped regularly in my San Francisco store, and he told me how he thought the term 'plastic food' must have originated. Some biochemist, he speculated, must have observed that, when looked at through a microscope, a hydrogenated fat molecule looks very much like a plastic molecule. Spontaneously, he or she coined the phrase.

"There was something in the conversation much more compelling to me than any notion he had about how the term originated. 'Well,' I asked, 'if it *looks* a lot like plastic, isn't it, in fact, a lot *like* plastic?'

'Yes,' he answered. 'Lipid chemists actually talk about *plasticizing* oils.'

"His answer made me think about what business I was in. I was selling a lot of margarine to people who were assuming, as I had, that it was real food. Should I just tell them about it, or should I take a more radical approach? I decided to discontinue selling margarine, as well as products containing vegetable shortening, margarine's cousin, and to perform a little experiment.

"It was a real layman's experiment, not the least bit technical. I put a cube of margarine, the kind I had been selling, on a saucer and placed the saucer on a windowsill in the back room of my store. I reasoned that if I made it readily available, and if it was real food, insects and microorganisms would invite themselves to the feast. Flies and ants and mold would be all over it, just as if it were butter. If nature treats this margarine the way it would treat butter, I thought, it would be circumstantial evidence that margarine is really more like food than like plastic. Seeing such evidence, I could then sell margarine again.

"That cube of margarine became infamous. I left it sitting on the windowsill for about two years. In all that time, nobody ever saw an insect of any description go near it. Not one speck of mold ever grew on it. All that ever happened was that it kind of half-puddled down from the heat of the sun beating through the windowpane, and it got dusty, very dusty. A cube of margarine doesn't clean up very well. Finally, it got to looking so revolting that I decided to terminate the experiment. For me, the experiment had not been foreshortened. I had reached the conclusion long before that margarine really is not food, that it's really a form of 'edible' plastic.

"Apart from the experiment, what brought me to that conclusion was learning about *hydrogenation,* the process of hardening vegetable oils so they can be made into margarine and vegetable shortening. Let's take a look at what happens in the process of hydrogenation, hardening the 'double bonds,' which link oil molecules together in 'chains.'

"Double bonds can be thought of as being like cracked links in a chain. A chain with a double bond, then, is not stiff; it tends to bend at every cracked link. Thus, it exhibits a lot of molecular activity. The more double bonds, that is, the more unsaturated, the more active the fatty acid molecule is.

"The stiff links of saturated fats are inactive and tend to stack up, creating a solid mass. Cracked links, on the other hand, keep the unsaturated molecules wriggling, tending to remain in the fluid state. Thus, an extremely polyunsaturated oil, like flax seed oil, will remain liquid even in the freezer.

"The only way a manufacturer can make margarine or vegetable shortening out of polyunsaturates—in other words, make a solid out of a liquid—is to deactivate the molecules by filling the cracks in the chain. That is the aim of *hydrogenation* and its sister process, *partial hydrogenation,* whether it is aimed at polyunsaturates (like safflower, soy, or corn oils), or monoun-saturates (like canola and peanut oils), or even saturates (like palm and coconut oils). No matter what kind of oil it is, hydrog-enation ruins its nutritional value.

"To hydrogenate, natural oils are heated under pressure for six to eight hours at 248–410 degrees F and reacted with hydro-gen gas, using a metal-like nickel or copper as a catalyst. If this process is brought to completion, as in vegetable shortening, you have a partially hardened oil, as in most margarines.

"In his book, *Fats and Oils,* Udo Erasmus refers to sat-urated vegetable oils as 'safe.' They are safe, he says, 'because they contain no trans fatty acids to interfere with essential fatty acid activity in the body. They are also 'safe' because they are dead, do not spoil, and therefore have a long shelf life. The problem with these 'safe' fats is that some of the altered molec-ular fragments formed in the process may be toxic, and the end product may be contaminated by traces of the metal catalyst.

"Nutritionally worse than saturated oils are the partially hardened fats produced by partial hydrogenation. This is due to the formation of *trans fatty* acids. In the natural, or *cis* form, double bonds have a pair of hydrogen atoms opposed to each other on opposite sides of the carbon chain. When partially hydrogenated, however, one of the hydrogens flips over to the other side. This transformation straightens the chain somewhat, making it a sort of imitation, half-baked saturate. According to *Bailey's Industrial Oil Guide,* the percentage of fat that has been transformed into trans fatty acids in margarines ranges between 20 percent and 40 percent. Erasmus says,

> Trans fatty acids compete for enzymes, produce biologically nonfunctional derivatives, and interfere with the work of the essential fatty acids in the body. Because of our association of the word "polyunsaturates" with health, we are fooled into thinking that we are buying a health-giving product of good quality, a product that is actually health-destroying.
>
> There are so many possibilities of different compounds that can be made during partial hydrogenation that they stagger

the imagination. Scientists have barely scratched the surface in studying all the changes induced in fats and oils by hydrogenation. Needless to say, the industry is hesitant to fund thorough and systematic studies on the kinds of chemicals produced and their effects on health. The industry is equally hesitant to publicize the information which already exists on the topic.

Two statements sum up the story of hydrogenation and health. The first statement, made by G. J. Bisson, Professor of Nutrition at Laval University in Quebec, says that "it would be practically impossible to predict with accuracy either the nature or the content of these new molecules (produced by hydrogenation). Between the parent vegetable oil sometimes labeled 'pure,' and the partially hydrogenated product, there is a world of chemistry that alters profoundly the composition and physiochemical properties of natural oils."

The other statement was made by Herbert Dutton, one of the oldest and most knowledgeable oil chemists in North America. It goes like this: "If the hydrogenation process were discovered today, it probably would not be adopted by the oil industry." He adds, "The basis for such comment lies in the recent awareness of our prior ignorance concerning the complexity of isomers formed during hydrogenation and their metabolic and physiological fates."

"If an altered fat molecule takes the place of an essential fat in your membrane structure, the result is that your membrane then has a faulty structure. What then? It depends on where the membrane is, what its purpose is, how many more of them there are—in any case, faulty structure causes a faulty function. Faulty membranes are just one of the many aberrations incorporated into natural defense systems by the altered molecules in our industrialized food supply.

"Hydrogenation, which until now has drawn so little attention, may turn out to be one of the very worst of the many nutritional insults introduced during the twentieth century. In the 1990s, death from heart attacks is thirty five times more frequent than it was in 1900. It would be foolish to suggest that hydrogenated fats are the sole cause of the contemporary epidemic of heart disease. But a little-known study undertaken in India suggests the major role played by altered fats in this tragic state of affairs. It was reported in the *American Journal of Clinical Nutrition,* 1967, 20: 462–75.

"The study was performed by Dr. Malhotra, medical doctor for the Indian National Rail System. He found two population groups in India, one in the north, the other in the south. The northerners were meat eaters, and the main source of fat in their diets was ghee (clarified butter). You might assume, therefore, that they had high cholesterol levels. You would be right.

"The southerners were vegetarians, with much lower cholesterol levels. Even so, they had *fifteen times* the rate of heart disease compared to their northern neighbors. The major dietary difference Dr. Malhotra found was in the kind of fat the southerners used. They had abandoned the traditional use of ghee— real food—in favor of 'plastic food'—margarine and refined polyunsaturated vegetable oils.

"A follow-up study done twenty years later found that the Indians in north India are now having many MI (heart attack) deaths. The British medical journal, *The Lancet* on November 14, 1987 contains a letter from Bihari S. Raheja of the Jaslok Hospital in Bombay. He wrote that MI deaths in India have greatly increased as the polyunsaturated liquid vegetable fats and the margarines made from them have largely replaced ghee in the Indian diet.

"It seemed there were two reasons for the switch: one was that margarine was cheaper than ghee; the other was that doctors had been telling people that they would be healthier if they replaced the 'bad' saturated fat of ghee with the 'good' polyunsaturated fat of refined vegetable oil. I wish I could tell those Indians not to believe it, that the modern experiment of replacing natural foods with industrialized foodstuffs has proved to be a health disaster. Maybe they would get the point if I could tell them about that cube of margarine, puddled miserably on a saucer on the windowsill of my back room in the late 60s in San Francisco."

&

CHAPTER 6

# Vegetable Oils: Their History, Properties, and Uses

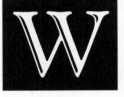

hich oil is best for sautéing? For baking? For salads? For mayonnaise?" Here are some simple guidelines. Generally, all unrefined oils have a lower smoke point, and therefore, are not recommended for high temperature frying. One exception is the high oleic sunflower and safflower oils. Both butter and ghee (clarified butter) are included in this section because, while they are not vegetable oils, they are excellent fats for cooking.

## Almond Oil

The almond tree has been cultivated in Asia for more than thirty five centuries. Unrefined almond oil is sweet and pleasant tasting and is known for its high content of vitamins A and E. It has long been used to beautify the skin, as an antiseptic for the intestines, and as a source of minerals. Almond oil is also used therapeutically in treating gastric ulcers and as a laxative, as well as to help stabilize the nervous system.

Making almond oil from food grade almonds is expensive, and very difficult to find in a cold-pressed form. Most almond oils on the market today are made from worm-eaten inedible nuts. Therefore, they are mostly used topically as massage oils or for treatment of burns.

## Borage Seed Oil

Borage seed oil was first used during the Middle Ages to insure good-quality blood. During the Renaissance, it was recommended as a cure for depression and to strengthen the heart. Borage seed oil is high in gamma linolenic acid, a derivative of the Omega-6 fatty acids, and has been used to help those with illnesses such as arthritis, allergies, multiple sclerosis, cancer, arteriosclerosis, immune system deficiency, diabetes, obesity, PMS, alcoholism, liver degeneration, colitis, depression, skin disorders, and other conditions.

Borage seed oil should only be used in small amounts, one-quarter to one-half teaspoon, one to two times daily. It can be taken by itself or on food. It should never be used in cooking and should be kept refrigerated. It also comes in capsules. Some companies are making a flax-borage seed oil combination capsule that provides an excellent balance of essential fatty acids with gamma linolenic acid. Borage seed oil contains twice as much GLA (gamma linolenic acid) as evening primrose oil.

## Butter

Butter has been used for thousands of years, and is good for any type of cooking. It is stable in the presence of light, heat, and oxygen. Nothing compares to the taste of butter. However, it is not high in essential fatty acids, so it should not be considered a source of these essential nutrients.

Used in moderation, the cholesterol content of butter should not be a problem if the diet has sufficient essential fatty acids, is free of poisonous fats, and contains those elements necessary for the efficient metabolism of fat. It is better to buy butter that is raw and unsalted, as it is a common practice with dairies to add salt to the old, rancid butter to disguise its taste and make it salable.

## Canola Oil

Canola is one of the most nutritious and best balanced oils. It is unique in that not only does it contain the Omega-9, -6 and -3 fatty acids in the unrefined organic state, but it is also a rich source of vitamin K, chlorophyll, beta carotene, and vitamin E.

Canola is a hybrid, derived from the mustard family. It dates back to antiquity in eastern Europe and Asia. It is used therapeutically to protect artery walls and as protection against blood clots. Recent strains of the plant contain less erucic acid than its ancestors, and the oil is gaining in popularity. Erucic acid in high amounts can be harmful.

Canola is a delicate oil with a rich, golden color and is best used directly on salads, raw vegetables, potatoes, grains, or cottage cheese. It has a light and delicate flavor, excellent in salad dressings and mayonnaise. Due to its Omega-3 fatty acid content, canola oil should not be used for cooking over 320 degrees F. Unrefined canola oil has a rich, strong flavor, and is wonderful as a fat replacement in bread recipes. I find both flax and canola delicious and use them on many dishes, often dipping bread or crackers in the oils in place of butter.

## Clarified Butter (Ghee)

Yvon Tremblay, a renowned French chef from Montreal, wrote the following about his use and appreciation of ghee or clarified butter.

> One of my favorite ways of cooking is to mix half ghee with half oil in preparing, marinating, or sauteing vegetables, fish, or meat. The taste is without compare, and the ghee will never burn if it is prepared properly. The smell of the ghee and oil cooking is exquisite and will have

such an effect on your guests that they will have to find out what has given your dish that special taste. This is one of the most treasured secrets of fine chefs. There are many reasons why the best chefs prefer ghee and the ghee–oil mixture for their cuisine.

• Ghee will never burn the dish you cook.

• It doesn't smoke, like butter, and develop toxic compounds if overheated.

• The aroma of one's cooking is completely different.

• It is good for coating pastries.

• Ghee is the most highly regarded cooking fat by two of the finest cuisines in the world, the French and the Indian.

Prepared ghee can be purchased in most health food stores and supermarkets. One can also make it using the following method:

Take 2 lbs of unsalted butter, cut into pieces, and place in a pot.

Using a low temperature, melt the butter until it is liquid and you can see the fat bubbling on top.

Cook on a low flame for 20 minutes. The impurities will rise to the top.

Place a piece of cheese cloth in a colander and strain the butter, or simply skim off the light-colored impurities and milk compounds from the top of the melted butter.

Ghee will keep much longer than butter and will store well even without refrigeration.

## Evening Primrose Oil

Evening primrose is similar to borage seed oil in that it has a high content of gamma linolenic acid. It also has been used to help people overcome PMS, allergies, arthritis, depression, skin disorders, colitis, multiple sclerosis, liver degeneration, alcoholism, cancer, arteriosclerosis, immune system weakness, obesity, and other disorders. Some tribes of Native Americans used the herb for asthma, skin disorders, and other conditions.

Evening primrose oil is a highly regarded therapeutic formula in Europe. Efamol—one of the major producers of evening primrose oil—has conducted full safety and efficacy trials in Europe. As a result, they have been granted licenses for the sale of pharmaceutical grade evening primrose oil in several countries including Great Britain, Ireland, Germany, Italy, Australia, and New Zealand. In addition, in Great Britain and Ireland, they have authorization to use the product for infants under two years of age, a positive demonstration of the oil's safety. Evening primrose oil is available in both liquid form and capsules.

## Flax Seed Oil

There is such extensive and valuable information on flax seed oil and flax meal that a chapter on each follows this one.

## Hazelnut Oil

The hazelnut is believed to have its origins in ancient Greece. Hazelnut oil has long been popular in finer European kitchens. The delicate flavor and bouquet of the hazelnut is exceptional on salads and pasta, and in pancakes, waffles, and muffins. Hazelnut oil is rich in monounsaturated fatty acids, similar to olive oil. Considered to be the finest gourmet cooking oil, it is preferred by many Gold Medal chefs for use in creating fine dishes and desserts.

Hazelnut oil is easily digested and high in minerals. Traditionally, it has been used in the treatment of parasites, tuberculosis, urinary disease, and colitis. It is recommended to people recovering from disease, the elderly, pregnant women, and diabetics. It is also an excellent oil to massage onto the skin.

## Olive Oil

According to Greek mythology, Poseidon and Athena were fighting over the most beautiful area in Greece. To avoid a conflict, it was decided that humans would choose a protecting god for themselves. To win their favor, Poseidon produced a marvelous horse. Athena brought an olive tree to the people. She won, and Athens was built in her honor.

Fresh olive oil has a wonderfully rich, aromatic bouquet. It is used therapeutically to nourish the liver and gall bladder, and is recommended for diabetics. Olive oil is high in monounsaturated fatty acids and is helpful in reducing cholesterol. It is also used topically for soothing burns, eczema, and psoriasis.

Olive oil has been used for centuries in Greek, French, and Italian cuisines, and gives even ordinary dishes a "Mediterranean" flavor. It is excellent for sautéing, makes a rich, exotic mayonnaise, and is delicious when used in salad dressings, sauces, and spreads.

However, most olive oil is neither properly made nor is it from organically grown olives. According to an article in *Consumer Reports,* October 1991, there are over ninety brands of olive oil sold in American markets or specialty stores. Words like "pure" and "light" are terms used for marketing strategies, without carefully defined standards. Imported "Extra Virgin" olive oil must meet European governmental rules for color, aroma, and flavor and must pass chemical tests. It must be hand harvested, and then spun in a centrifuge to separate the oil from the watery part. If the color and taste do not meet European standards of "perfect," the oil is called "Virgin" or "Superfine Virgin" (little of which is seen in the U.S.). Oil that does not meet these standards is called "pure" or, "less carefully culled fruit," and is refined, has solvents added, and is heated, leaving it colorless and flavorless (with 5 percent to 25 percent Extra Virgin oil added back). "Light" is refined, with even less Extra Virgin oil added back, with even less olive taste.[1]

At best, gourmet "Extra Virgin" olive oil, while meeting standards of color and flavor, is not organic. Also, the glass containers will allow light to penetrate possibly causing rancidity, and the metal ones can leach contaminants from the metal or solder. Omega Nutrition / Arrowhead Mills are the only companies that have third-party, certified organic olive oil packaged in light-excluding containers.

## Pistachio Nut Oil

Pistachio nut oil is an exquisite green oil with a rich, sweet taste. It has the most delicate taste of all the gourmet cooking oils, and is highly prized for the special flavor it lends to various dishes. It is composed of 10.9 percent palmitic acid, 54.1 percent oleic acid, and 30.4 percent linoleic acid.

## Pumpkin Seed Oil

Pumpkin seed or squash seed oil has been used throughout history in India, Europe, and the Americas. It has a good proportion of both the Omega-6 and Omega-3 essential fatty acids, making it one of the most nutritious oils. It is quite tasty and should not be cooked, but poured directly onto vegetables, pasta, and other dishes.

The seeds have similar properties, and are used to nourish and heal the digestive tract, fight parasites, improve circulation, help heal prostate disorders, and help prevent dental caries. Both the seeds and oil are recommended to pregnant and lactating women for their high essential fatty acid content.

A lack of certified organic pumpkin seeds has prevented the large scale production of this oil by the few reputable oil companies.

# Safflower Oil

The safflower, a member of the daisy family, is a native of the mountainous regions of southwest Asia and Ethiopia, and is grown extensively in India. This annual plant yields flowers, which are used in dye, and has oil-rich seeds. Safflower oil is a versatile vegetable oil. In its unrefined form, if manufactured correctly, it has a unique, wonderful flavor. It can be used for light sautéing, baking, stir-frying, and makes excellent dressings, sauces, dips, and mayonnaise. It is especially delicious in grain salads. Safflower oil is rich in polyunsaturated fatty acids.

# Sesame Oil

Sesame oil is the traditional oriental and macrobiotic cooking oil, providing the familiar sesame flavor in sautéed dishes. The sesame seed is a mainstay of nutrition in the Middle East, especially in Turkey. It is rich in lecithin, which helps build the nervous system and brain cells. It is used to help depression, stress, and improve circulation. It is also an excellent massage oil. In Ayurvedic medicine, sesame oil is prized for its soothing properties and is often used for foot massages for people who have a problem sleeping. A friend of mine claims great success with this therapy, especially after a transatlantic plane flight.

Sesame oil is rich in monounsaturated and polyunsaturated fatty acids, is very versatile, and can be used for all cooking needs. It also contains sesamol, a natural preservative, and is thus very stable. Sesame oil is a delicious ingredient for mayonnaise, dressings, spreads, and pasta toppings.

# Sunflower Oil

The sunflower originated in South America. The Incas, who worshipped the sun as their god, used its oil in many ways. It has a long history of being used to help the endocrine and nervous systems, and reduces cholesterol.

Sunflower oil gives the delicate nutty flavor of fresh sunflower seeds to salads, baked goods, and other dishes. It can be used for baking, light sautéing, and adds a wonderful flavor to salad dressings, sauces, and dips. It is rich in polyunsaturated fatty acids and vitamin E.

Several oils are included here separately:

## Black Currant Seed Oil

This is an interesting oil containing both Omega-3 and Omega-6 oils (including GLA and EPA, eicosapentaenoic acid). It is generated as a by-product of black currant jam or jelly. At this point, however, all commercial seeds from the jam companies are extracted with solvents and refined, leaving a questionable finished product, at best. Also, only seeds grown commercially with chemicals are currently available so, until more organic black currant jelly or jam is produced, we are not likely to see a quality version of this promising oil.

## Corn Oil

Due to the low oil content in corn, extremely high temperatures and toxic solvents are needed to extract the oil efficiently.

## Cottonseed Oil

Currently, there is very little organic cottonseed available. Cotton is one of the most heavily sprayed crops.

## Soy Oil

It is especially difficult to extract oil from soybeans. The soybeans must be roasted and treated by methods that damage the oil, and then subjected to further high temperatures and toxic solvents.

# Walnut Oil

Walnut oil has a delicious flavor, and is great to pour on salads or other dishes. Certain varieties of walnuts are excellent sources of the Omega-3 and Omega-6 fatty acids. However, all the walnut oils currently available in stores are heavily processed and refined, so they are not good to use. Omega Nutrition will manufacture fresh-pressed oil from organic walnuts for special orders.

# Avocado, Corn Germ, Grape Seed, Rice Bran, & Wheat Germ Oil

These are by-product oils. They are produced for the public primarily by companies that want an economic return from either 1) the discards or fiber that come from refining the grain, as in the case of corn, wheat, or rice, or 2) the remains from the wine pressing industry, as in the case of grapes, which would normally be sold either as livestock feed or composted. In some cases, these companies will even go as far as funding dubious research studies as part of an advertising campaign to lend validity to their oils.

While any seed oil will have some kind of nutritional value, the drawbacks of these oils are considerable. For one thing, the low oil content of the seed, hull, or germ, and/or the difficulty in extracting oil from varying consistencies of raw material, leads to the use of solvent extraction and heavy refining methods, primarily to create a marketable product.

For example, grape seed oil, in its raw form, is black in color and very strong tasting. Avocado oil is green and black, and very unpleasant tasting in its raw form. These oils require high temperature refining, creating trans fatty acids, free radicals, and other toxic substances.

Another concern is that the large majority of these products come from large commercial farms that make heavy use of chemical fertilizers, pesticides, and herbicides. The residues from pesticides and herbicides are often concentrated in the seed or outer bran, and can become concentrated in the oil.

## Tropical Oils: Palm, Palm Kernel, and Coconut

Palm oil, palm kernel, and coconut oils do not contain either of the essential Omega-6 or Omega-3 fatty acids to any appreciable degree, with the exception of palm oil, which contains 10 percent Omega-6. Their fats are easily digestible and function mostly as food for the body to use in energy production.

A few years ago, a successful campaign was carried out through the media to scare the American consumer away from "tropical oils." It claimed that the fat content of these oils contributed to heart disease, and that businesses and consumers should replace them with hydrogenated vegetable oils like soybean oil. This is an example of the results of well-meaning but misinformed spokespeople for our health.

Dr. C. Everett Koop, former Surgeon General of the United States, called the tropical oil scare "foolishness." "But to get the word to commercial interests terrorizing the public about nothing is another matter," he said.

As I have documented in this book, the problems of heart disease are manifold. Poisonous trans fats produced when unsaturated fats are subjected to refining and hydrogenation processes are much more implicated in causing arteriosclerosis than good quality saturated vegetable fats. There are also studies showing that good quality saturated fats from vegetable oils (none of which contain cholesterol), actually help to lower cholesterol and prevent heart disease.

## Palm Oil

Palm oil has been used for more than five thousand years, produced from the fleshy part of the palm fruit. It is the second-most produced oil in the world today. Annual production is 10.33

million tons, with soybean oil the largest at 15.04 million tons (of a total annual vegetable oil production of 77.33 million tons in 1989).

Palm oil is an interesting oil with many unique and beneficial properties. It is extracted solely by mechanical and physical methods without the use of poisonous solvents like hexane, commonly used to process other oils. In its crude form, it is among the richest sources of beta carotene and has a high content of vitamin E. Crude palm oil contains three hundred times more beta carotene than tomatoes and fifteen times more beta carotene than carrots. It has an interesting fatty acid profile, containing 40 percent Omega-9s (oleic acid-monosaturated), 44 percent palmitic acid (saturated), 10 percent Omega 6s (linoleic acid-unsaturated) and 5 percent stearic acid (saturated).

Many characteristics make palm oil desirable to use in manufactured food products. Its fatty acid composition gives it a desirable semi-solid consistency without needing hydrogenation. It is very resistant to oxidation and therefore has a good shelf life, holds up well in hot climates, and has properties making it excellent for use in cakes and bakery products. It is also readily available, and is inexpensive to produce compared to most other oils.

However, it is not currently recommended for use because only refined palm oil is available in North America and Europe. As usual, most of the vital nutrients are destroyed. Crude palm oil has a rich, reddish-brown color (which most consumers would probably reject). But the introduction of unrefined, organically grown palm oil, packaged in opaque containers, would be a valuable and nutritious product. Even as it exists now, though, it is better to use than other heavily refined, hydrogenated vegetable oils.

## Palm Kernel Oil

Palm kernel oil is extracted from the nut of the palm fruit. It is made up of saturated fat—51 percent lauric acid, 9 percent palmitic acid, 14 percent stearic acid, 18 percent myristic acid— and a small percentage of other fats. Its main advantage over other commercial oils, like palm oil, is that it is not subjected to hydrogenation in its processing methods, making it a purer oil.

## Coconut Oil

Coconut oil is composed of 90 percent of the medium chain tri-glyceride saturated fats. It is made up of 48 percent lauric acid, 17 percent myristic, 9 percent palmitic, 8 percent caprylic, 7 percent capric, 6 percent oleic, and a small percentage of several other fats. Coconut oil is excellent for cooking because of its heat resistant properties. Its fats are easily digested and metabolized and do not cause weight gain.

Besides food uses, it is also the primary fat used in making soap. If only it was available in an organically grown, unrefined state and packaged in light-excluding containers, we would have an excellent fat for cooking purposes.

## Cooking Methods

You may have noticed that we do not recommend any oil for use in deep-frying. The intense heat required for deep-frying destroys some of the properties of any oil, as well as creating poisonous compounds and toxic fatty acids. Therefore, this method of cooking is not recommended.

That does not mean, however, that oils should be eliminated altogether in cooking. Flavor and nutritional content can be enhanced with the proper use of oils. Wonderful combinations of vegetables, herbs, and spices, with tofu, nuts, or seeds added for variety, can be lightly sautéd in olive, hazelnut, sesame, safflower, or sunflower oil. The best fats for cooking are butter, ghee, olive, hazelnut, and sesame oil. Sunflower and safflower oil are delicate and should only be used for very light sautéing. Here is a basic recipe for sautéing:

Place 1–2 Tbs of oil in a frying pan, skillet, or wok. Heat the oil slowly over a low flame. Then, add ingredients according to the length of time needed to cook. (Denser, harder vegetables should go in first. Then, add the lighter vegetables, with leafy vegetables last). Stir often. An equal amount of butter or ghee can be added to the pan, making the delicious oil–butter or oil–ghee mixture.

If vegetables begin to stick, add ¼–½ cup of water, broth, or soup stock, and cover the pan. The steam from the liquid will cause the vegetables to cook quickly.

To turn the broth into a thick, delicious sauce, dissolve a teaspoon of arrowroot or kudzu in a small amount of cold water. Stir the mixture into the vegetables about a minute before they are finished.

ક્ર

1.  "Olive Oil," *Consumer Reports* (October, 1991): 667–668.

# CHAPTER 7

# The Wonder of
# Flax Seed Oil

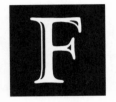lax is an ancient plant, highly prized by many civilizations for its nourishing and healing properties. Europeans, Native Americans, ancient Egyptians, among other cultures, used flax seed oil. Until the late 1800s and early 1900s, after which came the development of high technology and the mass production of refined oils, many towns and cities in Europe and North America still had small family-run workshops where they produced freshly made flax seed and other oils, and delivered them door-to-door, like the farmers who brought fresh milk.

The Cherokee Indians regarded flax as one of their most nourishing and healing herbs. They believed that flax seed oil captured energies from the sun that could be released and utilized in the body's life processes. This humble little plant was as sacred to them as the eagle feather.

They beat the seeds in a wooden funnel until the golden oil was freed from the shells and dripped into a waiting bowl. They used the oil by itself, or mixed it with curdled goat or moose milk (to form special lipoprotein compounds), honey and cooked pumpkin. The dish was used to nourish pregnant and nursing mothers to give them needed nutrients for creating strong and healthy children. It was also used to treat people who had skin diseases, arthritis, and malnutrition, and was given to men to increase their virility.

According to Dr. Johanna Budwig, mixing or blending flax seed oil with a good protein like raw, cultured, low-fat cottage cheese (similar to the Cherokees' dish) will provide even more nourishment. She has repeatedly observed that the flax seed oil and protein combination form special lipoprotein compounds that are easily digested. The body will use them to build new tissues. Dr. Budwig, Dr. Kousmine and other doctors in Europe use flax seed and other vegetable oils poured onto dishes or mixed with nonfat yogurt and/or cottage cheese as an essential part of their successful dietary therapies for cancer, heart disease, arteriosclerosis, arthritis, and many other modern maladies.[1,2,3]

People who have dairy allergies can use tofu, instead, or a high quality protein formula like the UltraClear, UltraBalance, or UltraMeal formulas distributed by Metagenics/Ethical Nutrients. Further information and specific recipes using flax seed oil and the flax seed oil-protein combinations are contained in chapter 12 of this book and *Healthful Cooking With Good Oils* by John Finnegan with Kathy Cituk, published by Elysian Arts.

Dr. Rudin and other authorities believe that a deficiency of the Omega-3 fatty acids has caused widespread illness, similar to preexisting conditions like scurvy (caused by a deficiency of vitamin C) and pellagra (caused by a deficiency of vitamin B3).[4,5,6]

One of the illnesses he feels to be the result of a deficiency of the Omega-3 fatty acids is depression, a major emotional disorder today. He and other doctors have successfully treated schizophrenia, depression, and other emotional disorders with a healthy diet, supplemented by one to two tablespoons per day of flax seed oil.[7,8]

While it is clear that people's estrangement from their true selves is the greatest cause of unhappiness today, there is no question that good nutrition also plays an essential role in our emotional health and well-being.

Besides being the most inexpensive and practical source of the Omega-3 fats, flax seed oil is also an excellent source of the Omega-6 fats, carotene, and vitamin E.

Athletes and fitness buffs find that using flax seed oil regularly, by itself, and in the oil-protein combination, greatly increases the oxygenation of their bodies, increases their stamina and improves their recovery time.

Many women find that the use of flax seed oil with a good diet and other nutritional support has prevented the development of stretch marks after having children.

There have been many scientific studies demonstrating the healing properties of flax seed oil:

- A research project in Australia used flax seed oil and linolenic acid to successfully fight strep infections in hospitals in Victoria.[9]
- A study done in Poland with rabbits observed that fatty acids, isolated from flax seed oil, exhibited a cell-destroying effect against certain cancer cells, with minimal destructive effect on the normal cells. After three hours, there was 100 percent destruction of carcinoma cells.[10]
- Flax seed oil has been used for decades as an essential part of therapies at the renowned Gerson Cancer Clinic.
- Several studies have found that the use of flax seed oil reduces pain, inflammation, and swelling caused by arthritis.[11]
- Flax seed oil has been found to lower high blood cholesterol and high triglyceride levels. It plays an essential role in softening and balancing the hardening effects of cholesterol in cellular membranes, and helps keep veins and arteries soft and pliable.[12]

&#1126;

1. Dr. Johanna Budwig, *Flax Oil as a True Aid Against Arthritis, Heart Infarction, Cancer and Other Diseases* (Vancouver, Canada: Apple Publishing, 1992).
2. Udo Erasmus, *Fats and Oils* (Canada: Alive, 1986).
3. William L. Fischer, *How to Fight Cancer and Win* (Canada: Alive, 1987).
4. Donald O. Rudin, M.D., and Clara Felix, *The Omega-3 Phenomenon* (New York: Rawson Associates, 1987).
5. Budwig, op. cit.
6. Dr. Randy L. Wysong, *Lipid Nutrition* (Michigan: Inquiry Press, 1990).
7. Rudin, op. cit.
8. Budwig, op. cit.
9. Fischer, op. cit.
10. Ibid.
11. Budwig, op. cit.
12. Ibid.

# CHAPTER 8

# Flax:
# The Friendly Fiber

**O**ur diets today contain less than one-third the fiber than either our grandparents had, or people who live in more rural areas of the world have. The average Western diet contains ten to twenty grams per day of dietary fiber, while the diets of most rural societies contain forty to sixty grams per day. According to the now classic paper by Dr. Denis Burkitt, published in *The Lancet* in 1969, entitled "Related Diseases—Related Cause?", the intestinal diseases which are prevalent throughout civilized nations are almost unknown in rural Africa and many other societies.

According to Dr. Burkitt, most leading degenerative diseases are partially caused by an insufficient intake of dietary fiber. These diseases include coronary heart disease, diverticular disease, appendicitis, hemorrhoids, varicose veins, obesity, and diabetes. The second most common cause of death from cancer is cancer of the colon, which has been firmly linked to a low fiber diet. Even Candida overgrowth is associated with low fiber diets. And recently, we have seen a spate of articles about using oat bran to reduce cholesterol. Although this information is just now receiving attention from the media, nutritional healers have been saying these things for decades.

There are five known functions that fiber performs:

1. Reduces intestinal toxicity and pathogenic bacterial and yeast overgrowth.

2. Improves bowel functioning and transit time.

3. Stabilizes blood sugar. Many medical tests have shown that fiber helps regulate both diabetes and hypoglycemia.

4. Lowers cholesterol.

5. Protects against other chronic degenerative diseases, such as cancer of the colon, hemorrhoids, and varicose veins. Proper use of fiber has been firmly established as the most effective therapy for hemorrhoids.

There are several ways to improve your dietary intake of good quality fiber. Reduce consumption of overly refined foods. Eat a salad every day with plenty of lettuce, grated carrot, and other fibrous vegetables. Use a liberal amount of whole grains and legumes in your diet. And, when needed, take a high quality fiber supplement.

There is much media attention on the topic of fiber. But all the terminology—words like "soluble" and "insoluble"—can leave the consumer baffled. There are at least eight different kinds of dietary fiber. Dietary fiber is plant cells that are not digested by the human system. They are broken down into two categories:

1. *Soluble fibers,* which include pectins, gums, mucilage, and sterols.

2. *Insoluble fibers,* which include celluloses, hemicelluloses, lignins, and waxes.

Insoluble fibers are an irritant to the colon and are used as a laxative. Wheat bran is the most commonly used. Soluble fibers form a jellylike mass, gently regulating the flow of fecal matter through the colon and dissolving any hardened material lining the colon walls. Flax, psyllium, and oat bran are most commonly used for this purpose. They help both constipation and diarrhea, depending on the amount of water you consume.

Both fibers, soluble and insoluble, play an important role in the prevention of constipation, colon cancer, gall and kidney stones, colitis, diverticulitis, and heart disease. They also aid in the dietary control of diabetes, and increase fertility. Few foods contain both types of fibers. Flax and prunes are the best, with the fiber from flax being at the top of the list.

Besides being a well-rounded source of both the fibers, flax contains another component called lignans (not to be confused with lignins). Lignans are compounds found in some higher plants which have attracted the attention of the research community.

Lignans have anticancer, antibacterial, antifungal, and antiviral properties. Plant lignans are the dietary precursors to several kinds of human lignans formed in the intestinal tract by bacteria from fiber-rich food. These lignans have been isolated and studied at the University of Toronto and other research facilities. They found that lignans, in the presence of beneficial flora in the human intestine, form very potent anticancer substances, particularly against the hormone-driven cancers such as breast, colon, prostate, uterine, and ovarian.[1,2]

The flax lignan is a glucoside which produces enterolactone and enterodiol in people. Enterolactone is, quantitatively, the most important animal lignan. These lignans have a structure resembling synthetic estrogens, but have antiestrogenic properties, a dietary action associated with protection against colon and breast cancer.

Organic flax seed is, by far, the richest source of the valuable plant lignan. Wheat also contains many lignans, but flax has over one hundred times more. Other major sources, such as rye, buckwheat, millet, soy, oat, and barley yield two to six micrograms of lignans per gram of grain, while ground flax seed yields an extraordinary eight hundred micrograms per gram.

Flax fiber is also very tasty. It mixes well with one-half apple juice and one-half water. It should be noted that flax does absorb seven times its weight in water so one should be sure to consume adequate water when taking it. Flax promotes excellent colon health. Choosing a flax fiber can be difficult for several reasons. If you simply grind the seed and try to eat it, you will encounter several problems:

1.  Because of the high content of fragile Omega-3 fatty acids, exposure to light and oxygen will begin oxidation and free radical activity. It should be eaten within fifteen minutes of being ground.

2.  Because of enzyme inhibitors found in all raw nuts, seeds, and grains, one could experience digestive upset (similar to when one eats raw dough or nuts), although it is still not proven whether there are enough enzyme inhibitors in fresh ground flax meal to be harmful to the average person.

3.  There are B6 inhibitors in flax.

4.  There are pesticide and herbicide residues in commercial flax.

One company has solved all these problems and has an exceptional organic flax fiber called Nutri-Flax sold under the Arrowhead label and the Omega Nutrition label. Omega Nutrition makes their fiber in a similar way to how they make their high quality flax seed oil. Their fiber is low-fat (only 13 percent fat in Nutri-Flax, compared to 40 percent in the whole seed), and is warmed slightly to inactivate enzyme inhibitors, but keep beneficial enzymes intact. They add B6, zinc, and natural vitamin E. Packaged in a light-proof, oxygen-free container, it provides the consumer with an easy to take, good-tasting product.

Psyllium is the most widely consumed fiber today, the main ingredient of intestinal cleansers in health food markets, and in products like Metamucil, which dominate the geriatric market. However, there are several problems with psyllium. There is no organic psyllium available, partly because containers have to be irradiated prior to leaving India—where it is grown—to kill bacteria and bugs. All psyllium entering Canada is treated with ethylene oxide to kill bugs and pests. All psyllium entering the

U.S. is either irradiated or treated with a gaseous bromine compound (a pesticide) to kill insects. (Bromine is a vile substance with residuals like fluorine and chlorine.) Psyllium also has very little nutritional value, contains no beneficial lignans, and is like trying to swallow gelatin.

Flax fiber (at least Nutri-Flax) is organic, contains 36 percent protein, a wide range of minerals, has a nutty flavor, and contains valuable lignans. To get the anticancer effect from flax meal, one teaspoon a day is all that is required. Colon cleansing after a fast will require several tablespoons a day. When choosing a flax fiber, make sure it meets the criteria mentioned earlier.

At one time, flax was believed to have cyanogenic glycosides (a form of cyanide), but this exists only in certain varieties of the raw seed. The product from Omega Nutrition is gently warmed to inactivate the cyanogenic glycosides, and tests free of it.

The breakdown of flax seed meal fat content is: 7 percent Omega-3s, 16 percent Omega-6s, and 18 percent Omega-9s. It also contains 37 percent high quality protein, 35 percent carbohydrates, and 37 percent total fiber, composed of 60 percent insoluble fiber and 40 percent soluble fiber.

Flax seed meal has an excellent composition of vitamins and minerals, including calcium, magnesium, zinc, iron, manganese, phosphate, pantothenic acid, niacin, riboflavin, and thiamin. It also contains a healthy amount of beta carotene.

Flax seed meal has a high mucilage content. This combination of high lignans, fiber, and essential fatty acid content makes it very healing for the lining of the digestive tract, for irritable bowel syndrome, and for inflamed bowel conditions.

One woman I know who was raised on a farm said that they regularly fed fresh-ground flax meal to their cows and horses whenever they developed digestive disorders like diarrhea, and also fed it to them to improve their coats. Several studies with young chickens and cows have shown that inclusion of flax seed meal in their diets resulted in a substantial increase in their weight and growth.

Another striking study that has just been released shows the effectiveness of flax seed oil and flax seed meal in combating malaria.[3,4,5] In many parts of the world, malaria is increasing in epidemic proportions. There are no known practical, cost-effective measures to contain it. According to a report by the U.S. National Academy of Sciences, Institute of Medicine, the outlook for malarial control is grim.

Before the development of quinine and the widespread application of DDT, malaria was the most infectious disease in the world, at times killing tens of millions each year. Now the malaria parasite has developed a resistance to quinine, and, once again, it is becoming increasingly difficult to effectively combat. Interestingly, the whole herb, Peruvian bark, is still effective against malaria, while the synthetic medicine of just one of its active ingredients is no longer effective. This is a powerful example of the difference in effectiveness and importance of whole herbal extracts as opposed to synthesized, isolated ingredients. But that is a topic for discussion in another book.

These studies, showing the effectiveness of flax seed oil and flax seed meal against cancer, malaria, heart disease, colitis, and many other conditions, deserve the consideration of all medical practitioners and anyone seriously concerned with maintaining their health and the health of their families.

1.  L. Thompson and M. Serrino, "Lignans in Flax Seed and Breast and Colon Carcogensis," Department of Nutritional Sciences, University of Toronto, Ontario, Canada.
2.  H. Aldercreutz, "Does fiber-rich food containing animal lignan precursers protect against both colon and breast cancer? An extension of the 'fiber hypothesis.'" *Gastrenterol* 86 (1984): 761–6.
3.  O.A. Levander, Al.L. Ager, V.C. Morris and R.G. May, "Protective effect of linseed oil against malaria vitamin E-deficient mice." Flax Inst. of the U.S., Proc. 53 (1990): 16–19.
4.  O.A. Levander, Al.L. Ager, V.C. Morris and R.G. May, "Protective effect of ground flax seed or ethyl linolenate in a vitamin E-deficient diet against murine malaria," *Nutr. Res.* 11 (1991): 941–48.
5.  O.A. Levander, Al.L. Ager, V.C. Morris, R. Fontela and R.G. May, "Suppression of malaria by dietary oxidant stress." Proc. 5th Int. Congress on Oxygen Radicals (Kyoto, Japan, in press, 1992).

CHAPTER 9

# The Oil-Protein Combination

T he Cherokee Indians were the first people known to have developed a special lipoprotein (oil-protein) food, combining flax seed oil, cultured cottage cheese, honey, and pumpkin to heal degenerative diseases and to build up strength and muscle tissue. Dr. Johanna Budwig developed a similar lipoprotein formula in her work to heal people with degenerative diseases. The crucial role that lipo-proteins play in maintaining our health deserves further exam-ination; the implications of this discovery are far-reaching.

Dr. Budwig came to her conclusions after a great deal of meticulous research and study. She analyzed thousands of blood samples from people who were healthy and people who were ill. She discovered that healthy people contained ample amounts of the essential fatty acids and sulphur-rich proteins in their blood and tissues, whereas people with illnesses were deficient in these vital lipoprotein substances. She also discovered that these lipo-proteins play a critical part in many key biochemical processes. They are an essential component in the body's oxygen-transport mechanisms and in the creation of hemoglobin. They are also the main substance used to build the membranes in each and every cell and, as such, enhance our bodies' ability to resist and fight disease-causing viruses, bacteria, yeasts, and parasites.

Once Dr. Budwig witnessed the important function of the lipoproteins, she reasoned that giving these compounds to patients should greatly aid in their recovery. She then searched for the best sources of complete protein and Omega-6 and Omega-3 fatty acids and decided that skim milk mixed with fresh-pressed flax seed oil offered the best source of the lipoprotein combination. She fed patients mixtures of one hundred grams of skim milk with forty grams of flax seed oil and twenty five grams of milk. (She now uses low-fat cultured cottage cheese instead of skim milk.) Within days, their energy began to return, their skin color improved, and they began to gain weight. Those with shallow breathing found that they could breathe more easily and that their body temperatures rose as their metabolism increased. Over a period of several months, Dr. Budwig found that her patients' tumors shrank and disappeared, and that liver dysfunction, atherosclerosis, and anemia all showed substantial improvement.

Sick and weak bodies have difficulty digesting, assimilating, and metabolizing food. The process of breaking down, assimilating, and recombining fats and proteins in their separate forms is easy for healthy people, but difficult for those with serious illnesses. This is one reason why it is so important to give them the premade lipoprotein mixture. Their bodies utilize it far easier than separate fats and proteins.

Of course, the flax seed oil / cottage cheese recipe was only part of her therapeutic program. She also put people on a high quality diet consisting entirely of organic foods, including buckwheat, potatoes, fresh fruits and vegetables, nuts and seeds, rainbow trout, fresh-pressed organic fruit and vegetable juices, herbal teas, and plenty of flax seed meal. She advised them to use additional amounts of sunflower, thistle, walnut, pumpkin seed, and other oils, which provide a complement of the Omega-6 fatty acids. Finally, she had people massage their bodies with a special blend of oils several times a week.

The above is a simplified explanation of Dr. Budwig's theory. She has many other interesting insights, such as the postulate that the Omega-3 and Omega-6 fats are high electron donors which release energy, directly feeding the heart muscle and all the cells in the body. Most of her books are published only in German and have not yet been translated. The best explanations of her research are presented in *How to Fight Cancer and Win* by William Fischer and *Fats and Oils* by Udo Erasmus, both published by Alive Books. Recently, a small publication of her work was released in English, *Flax Oil as a True Aid against Arthritis, Heart Infarction, Cancer, and Other Diseases* by Apple Publishing in Vancouver, British Columbia, but is now out of print.

What is known for certain is that the essential Omega-3 and -6 essential fatty acids and sulphur proteins are vital to maintain our good health and to fight disease, and lipoprotein compounds are easier to digest and assimilate than fats by themselves.

People who have allergies to dairy products can blend the flax seed oil into soy milk or tofu to produce the lipoprotein formula. For those allergic to soy as well as dairy products, Jeffrey Bland, Ph.D., has developed UltraClear. An exceptional formula, it uses a hypoallergenic, processed white rice as a protein source in its base which I mix with flax seed oil and flax seed meal. This formula is distributed by Metagenics and contains a full complement of high quality carbohydrates, vitamins, minerals, and antioxidants. It is used with great success in detoxification programs for many conditions, including Chronic Fatigue Syndrome, Candidiasis, the universal allergic syndrome, liver disorders, gastrointestinal disorders, and other conditions. I have been working with flax seed oil-protein formulas for some time with excellent results.

Most people I have worked with who are ill also had dairy allergies. I have developed special smoothie formulas using Ultra-Clear or UltraBalance as a base, adding different blends of the Omega-3 and -6 fats, flax seed meal, Chinese herbs, enzymes, and other rejuvenating substances. My forthcoming oils cookbook and weight management books present many recipes using the oil-protein combination.

Here is the story told by my friend Sandy, who gives her firsthand account of the powerful oil-protein combination.

# Sandy

"At the age of 30, I felt I was in poor health. At the urging of friends, I went to see a holistic health counselor in Boulder, Colorado. He told me that every organ in my body was in extremely poor condition. He suggested a comprehensive dietary and lifestyle program.

"I followed the health program faithfully, but still had lingering problems. After listing these problems, I was amazed to see that they matched almost all the symptoms listed as Omega-3 and Omega-6 fatty acid deficiencies described in Udo Erasmus' book *Fats and Oils,* John Finnegan's book *The Facts About Fats,* and other fats and oils literature. They were:

- eczema and other skin rashes
- wounds and infections healing slowly or not at all
- lingering immune system sensitivities
- chronic liver problems including jaundice
- arthritis-like symptoms
- increasing heart and circulatory problems—capillaries and occasionally larger blood vessels collapsing or breaking very easily. Irregularity of heart beat.
- tingling and numbness in arms, legs, and at times, throughout the body

"When I read Dr. Budwig's explanation of how sulphur-bound amino acids combine with fatty acids to form new cell membranes after a cell divided into two, I realized that for a long time, I had only gotten very tiny amounts of Omega-3 or none at all. I was probably stripping my body of the materials it needed to create new cells. Even the Omega-6 I got from more than a teaspoon of sesame seeds produced congestion and mucus in my lungs and nasal passages, and skin blemishes. My body was barely using the small amount of good fats I took in. I was like the starved dog whose condition was worsened by being given fats alone or protein alone but who managed to survive without either. I never thought to combine the two!

"I realized that I should try combining flax oil with sulphur-rich protein. Since I was dairy sensitive, milk was out of the question. I experimented and found that using soy milk, either ground sesame, sunflower, or flax seeds, and the whole grain quinoa in a cereal provided excellent amounts of amino acids. I added a tablespoon of flax oil to the mixture and some raisins on the cereal.

"For the last several months I have followed my usual diet of organically grown whole grains, vegetables, beans, sea vegetables, seeds, fruit, a few nuts and free-range chicken once a week. To this diet, I have added daily: 1 to 2 Tbsp. of flax oil, 1 to 2 Tbsp. ground flax seed salt, 1 to 2 Tbsp. of ground sesame or sunflower seeds, and the soy milk-cereal combination every other day or so. I also take 1 capsule of borage oil. When there is an inability of the body to produce GLA from the Omega-6 fatty acids, borage oil, which contains GLA, can supply this to the body directly.

"The changes I have noticed so far have been very encouraging. The first change was a disappearance of the stubborn eczema that had bothered me for years. There was an immediate increase in my ability to utilize good fats, increasing my intake to 3 to 4 Tbsp. daily without any mucus or congestion. The sense that my tissues and muscles could easily tear has been replaced by a feeling of strength and resilience. I have felt an increase in energy and mental clarity. I have noticed less sensitivity to environmental toxins. My tendency to jaundice has been steadily improving. The little moles on my body, including several on my head, have begun to shrink. The little lump in my breast and the one in my abdomen have become softer and smaller. Usually I would have to eat very small amounts of protein and fat to keep these lumps from growing. And the green color in different parts of my body has changed back to the natural color." (Budwig and other medical researchers have linked this greenish color with degenerative health and the development of cancerous conditions.) "I am now recommending whole fresh ground organic sesame, sunflower, and flax seeds and their unrefined oils in combination with sulphur-bound proteins to all my friends!"

# Culinary Uses of Fresh Pressed Organic Vegetable Oils

| Type of Oils | *Prepared Foods | Salads | Baking | Light Sautéing |
|---|:---:|:---:|:---:|:---:|
| Almond | * | * | * | * |
| Canola | * | * | | |
| Flax | * | * | | |
| Hazelnut | * | * | * | * |
| Olive | * | * | * | * |
| Pistachio | * | * | | |
| Pumpkin | * | * | | |
| Safflower | * | * | * | |
| Sesame | * | * | * | * |
| Sunflower | * | * | * | |
| Walnut | * | * | | |

We do not recommend high temperature frying or deep frying for healthful use of oils.

*Prepared Foods—in this category we are indicating to add these oils *after* the food has been cooked.

© 1992 John Finnegan

# Fatty Acid Profile for Fresh Pressed Organic Vegetable Oils

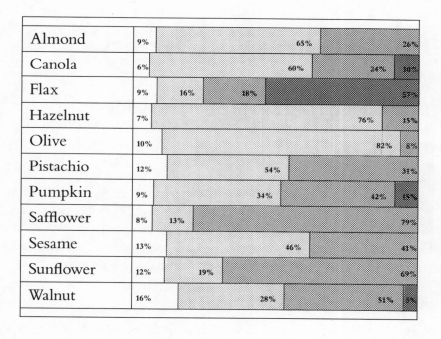

| Oil | | | | |
|-----|-----|-----|-----|-----|
| Almond | 9% | 65% | 26% | |
| Canola | 6% | 60% | 24% | 10% |
| Flax | 9% | 16% | 18% | 57% |
| Hazelnut | 7% | 76% | 15% | |
| Olive | 10% | 82% | 8% | |
| Pistachio | 12% | 54% | 31% | |
| Pumpkin | 9% | 34% | 42% | 15% |
| Safflower | 8% | 13% | 79% | |
| Sesame | 13% | 46% | 41% | |
| Sunflower | 12% | 19% | 69% | |
| Walnut | 16% | 28% | 51% | 5% |

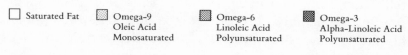

☐ Saturated Fat     Omega-9
Oleic Acid
Monosaturated     Omega-6
Linoleic Acid
Polyunsaturated     Omega-3
Alpha-Linoleic Acid
Polyunsaturated

© 1992 John Finnegan

# CHAPTER 10

# Essential Fatty Acids in Health and Disease

## The Functions of Essential Fatty Acids

The Omega-3 and Omega-6 essential fatty acids are nutrients vital to nearly all bodily processes. They nourish the body and help prevent and heal many conditions. Following is a list of these conditions and the ways in which the essential fatty acids work on them.

### Alcoholism and Addictions

A number of studies have found that alcoholics and addicts are usually deficient in Omega-3 fatty acids and consequently, certain prostaglandins. Use of flax seed oil and gamma linolenic acid (GLA) have substantially reduced depression and withdrawal symptoms and greatly aided recovery.[1,2] Omega-3 and Omega-6 fatty acids and GLA provide the necessary raw materials for the body to make prostaglandins. This is an important aspect of the recovering alcoholic's program for several reasons.

Firstly, a deficiency in needed prostaglandins can be a major metabolic factor causing the mental-emotional depression

and imbalance that often leads to a craving for addictive substances. Use of gamma linolenic acid will help correct this biochemical malfunction.

Secondly, preliminary tests in humans have shown that
gamma linolenic acid can make withdrawal from alcohol easier,
and can relieve postdrinking depression.[3] Dr. John Rotrosen and
Dr. David Sagarnick at New York University did similar tests
on mice. They addicted mice to alcohol by giving them an
alcohol-rich diet. Then they took away the alcohol abruptly.
Over the next few hours, the mice experienced dramatic withdrawal symptoms, similar to what happens with human alcoholics. The doctors then injected PGE1 (prostaglandins series 1)
into the animals. This dramatically alleviated the withdrawal
symptoms in the addicted mice. Tremor, irritability, overex-
citability, and convulsions were all reduced by about 50 percent.[4]
Gamma linolenic acid had the same effect as PGE1 in preventing
withdrawal symptoms.

Thirdly, gamma linolenic acid has shown significant effects
in healing liver damage caused by alcohol abuse. A very recent
study done at the Alcoholic Clinic at Craig Dunaine Hospital in
Inverness, Scotland showed that gamma linolenic acid can be
very helpful in correcting liver damage due to alcohol.

Under consultant psychiatrist Dr. Iain Glen, the clinic
conducted a double-blind trial with approximately one hundred
patients. No one knew who was taking capsules of gamma
linolenic acid, and who was taking identical capsules containing
liquid paraffin (a placebo).

The group who took evening primrose oil as a source of
GLA did much better than the other group. The results showed
that GLA can improve liver function, reduce the demand for
tranquilizers, improve brain function, and lower the incidence of
hallucinations during the period of alcohol withdrawal. The
liver, in particular, seemed to benefit. Its biochemistry returned
to normal much more rapidly among the patients taking gamma
linolenic acid.

Dr. Glen has worked on the hypothesis that drinking can seriously alter the body's membrane lipids. When he delivered his paper to an International Conference on "Pharmacological Treatments for Alcoholism" in London, March 1983, he commented:

> We used evening primrose oil because it contains a large amount of gamma linolenic acid. These membrane changes can block the linolenic acid metabolism. So, by giving alcoholics capsules of *Efamol* (a brand of evening primrose oil), we hoped to bypass this trouble. *Efamol* is the first specific medicine to show promise in treating alcohol dependence.[5,6]

Since then, researchers have discovered that borage seed oil has twice as much GLA as evening primrose oil. They have also found that giving people flax seed oil as well, provides the body with the necessary building blocks for it to make other important prostaglandins.

In one of the most recent books to date on this subject, *Essential Fatty Acids and Immunity in Mental Health,* Charles Bates, Ph.D., describes the cases of many recovering alcoholics who are greatly aided by the use of gamma linolenic acid. He found that some people have an inability to convert Omega-6 fatty acids into the essential PGE1 and PGE2 prostaglandins series. This is further compounded by the fact that most people also have excessive amounts of poisonous trans fatty acids and serious deficiencies of the Omega-3 and PGE 3 prostaglandins series.

What Bates found is that the PGE1 and PGE2 prostaglandins deficiency caused chronic depression and fatigue, but that drinking alcohol caused a temporary increase in the release of prostaglandins, alleviating the depression and fatigue. The effect was only temporary; later, the conditions worsened. Gamma linolenic acid increased the manufacture of the PGE1 and PGE2 prostaglandins series. The depression and fatigue cleared up, and most of the craving for alcohol disappeared.

# Allergies

One of the causes of allergies is leaky cell membranes. Omega-3 fatty acids and gamma linolenic acid help normalize allergic and inflammatory reactions. Recently, I was speaking with a young woman who grew up on a farm outside of Zurich, Switzerland. She told me that in twenty years of living in Switzerland, she had never known a single person who had allergies. Yet here, in the U.S., almost everyone she meets has allergies to either foods or inhalant substances. Observations like these lend credence to our theories that the current breakdown of people's health and immune system function is the result of changes in our diets and foods, and toxins in our air, food, and water.

# Allergies (Food )

One of the most thorough and up-to-date books on the relation-ship between food allergies and essential fatty acid and prosta-glandin deficiencies is *Essential Fatty Acids and Immunity in Mental Health* by Dr. Bates.

Since EFAs are the main building blocks of all cellular membranes in the human body, a deficiency can cause excessive permeability and irritability in both the digestive tract and the brain.[7,8,9] A deficiency of the PGE1—which is derived from the Omega-6 fatty acid—in the GI tract, creates low mucus secre-tion, high levels of gastric acid, and excessive inflammatory histamine. GLA and flax seed oil, taken with meals, often brings about marked improvement in those afflicted with food allergies, as well as allergies in general.[10]

# Anemia

A deficiency of Omega-6 fatty acids is the cause of one form of anemia. The lipoproteins of the blood are made from the phos-phatides containing Omega-6s, combined with sulphur-rich pro-teins. These lipoproteins are a key component of hemoglobin, the blood's oxygen carrier, and when insufficient, the blood becomes anemic.[11]

## Arthritis

Omega-3 fatty acids and GLA have often helped improve arthritic conditions. A double-blind, placebo-controlled study in England tested the effects of taking a combination of evening primrose and fish oil for rheumatoid arthritis. The study found that 60 percent of the patients receiving this oil combination were able to completely discontinue their nonsteroidal anti-inflammatory drugs. Another 20 percent were able to cut their dose of these drugs in half. The final 20 percent reported improvements, but maintained their drug dose. When the oil was replaced by a placebo, all patients deteriorated again within three months. The researcher concluded: "This opens a completely new treatment for rheumatoid arthritis."[12]

## Cancer

Omega-3 fatty acids have been found to help prevent and cure cancer. In 1986, the *Journal of the National Cancer Institute* printed a study that shows that alpha-linolenic acid kills human cancer cells in tissue culture without harming the normal cells.[13]

Dr. Johanna Budwig has documented many recoveries from cancer by prescribing a good diet supplemented with high quality flax seed oil.[14,15] In her search for an underlying cause and cure of cancer, heart disease, and other modern diseases, Dr. Budwig analyzed blood samples from people healthy and ill. Her research revealed that blood samples from people who had cancer, diabetes, and some kinds of liver disease consistently lacked the Omega-3 fatty acid. The blood samples also were found to lack the phosphatides, a substance necessary for the development and integrity of cellular membranes. Interestingly, the Omega-3 and Omega-6 fatty acids are a critical component of the phosphatides.[16]

In 1988, a study in the *Journal of the American Oil Chemists Society* reported that rats with implanted tumors who were fed flax seed oil, got fewer and smaller tumors, less metastasis, and had longer survival time than rats who were given corn oil instead.[17]

Also in 1988, the Linus Pauling Institute of Science and

Medicine fed tumor-prone mice one of five different refined fats and studied the rate of spontaneous tumor formation. Mice that were fed flax seed oil produced two spontaneous tumors. Those fed fish oil produced six. Mice fed lard (saturated) produced thirty two tumors. Those fed corn oil produced sixty tumors, and those fed safflower produced sixty six.[18] This study shows both the importance of having a balance of Omega-3 and Omega-6 fats, and of using unrefined oils in the prevention and treatment of cancer. All the oils that were refined and did not have a balance of both of these fats and GLA (gamma linolenic acid), enhanced tumor growth.

Nobel Prize winner Dr. Warburg has shown in an often duplicated test that healthy human cells will become cancerous when deprived of oxygen. From one perspective, cancer cells are simply undeveloped cells that use an anaerobic respiration process instead of an aerobic respiration process. This inability of the cells to fully develop may be caused by an absence of the key materials the cells use to create their membranes. Their respiration process becomes anaerobic because of an absence of the essential nutrients needed for an aerobic respiratory process.

## Cancer (skin)

One of the causes of skin cancer is the destruction of the ozone layer, but there are many other factors to be considered, as well.

1. Deficiencies of essential nutrients and the accumulation of poisons from food, water, and air are all factors.
2. Since essential fats are the main components of cellular membranes, one of the main protective factors of the entire surface of the skin is the composition and the quality of the fats that make up the skin.
3. The consumption of refined and hydrogenated oils and the deficiency of the Omega-3 fats is, without question, a major cause of skin cancer.

## Candida

Another widespread illness related to the Omega-3 deficiency and the consumption of toxic, processed oils, is Candida. One of the main causes of the development of Candida overgrowth in the digestive tract is a breakdown in the integrity of the tissues lining the stomach and intestinal walls. This has several detrimental effects. It enables poisons from the digestive tract and Candida secretions to penetrate through the lining into the bloodstream. These poisons will then circulate through the body, causing everything from allergies to depression and a susceptibility to staph infections.

In a normal, healthy person, the Candida and related species of yeast, controlled by the beneficial digestive flora, are benign and do not infect the host. When a person's flora is altered—either through the use of antibiotics and other medications, or when one becomes seriously malnourished and deficient in the Omega-3 fatty acids and other vital nutrients—the normally benign yeast changes into an aggressive form and, from starvation, attacks the walls of the digestive tract in the search for proper nourishment.

Malnutrition not only causes illness by nutrient deficiencies, it also has a profound, but not generally known effect. It creates a weakened organism, making it susceptible to many forms of latent bacteria, parasites, yeasts, and viruses which assault and devour the host. Not a pretty picture. The importance of eating well must be better understood by modern societies.

## Cellular Membranes: Strengthens the Integrity of the Cellular Membranes

Essential fatty acids are the major constituent of all cellular membranes in the body. Maintaining the integrity of these membranes helps prevent infection by yeasts, viruses, bacteria, and parasites. EFAs hold proteins in the membrane by the electrostatic attractive force of their double bonds and are involved in the traffic of substances in and out of the cells via protein channels, pumps, and other special mechanisms.[19,20,21]

One major cause of breakdown in the immune system is an overall weakening in cellular membrane integrity. The cells in the walls of healthy cells have the ability to discriminate between what to allow in and what to keep out. In other words, they can resist entry by viruses and other pathogenic agents and, at the same time, facilitate the entry of nutrients. This cellular membrane capacity—to recognize what is beneficial to its health and keep out the rest—is vital to our immune system and our basic strength, health, and functioning. When we consider that all the surfaces of our skin, digestive tract, mouth, sinuses, and throat are covered with trillions of bacteria, viruses, parasites, and yeasts, and even one square inch has millions of these creatures, a cell's ability to recognize and keep out those that are pathogenic is critical to the survival of the host. It is interesting to note that there have been many experiments in which healthy people were inoculated with living cancer viruses, and yet failed to become ill.

This suggests that a breakdown in the strength of the immune system is taking place among the populations of the industrialized nations, and the weakening of the discrimination and resistance of our cellular membranes is contributing to it. This leads us to ask, what changes are causing this deterioration?

Think of your cell walls as the walls of a house. If the walls of your house are made with bricks and mortar of good quality ingredients, mixed in the proper proportions, you will have a strong house. It will keep out the wind, rain, snow, cold, and insects. But suppose some of the key ingredients of these bricks and mortar are missing, in some cases replaced by inferior ingredients? The walls of your house will then be vulnerable to the elements and may crumble and fall.

A recent scandal in the United States exposed certain bolt manufacturers who, for several decades, cut corners. They made bolts out of inferior metals, but claimed they were of better quality. Lives were lost in numerous accidents as bridges collapsed and army vehicles broke down when the cheap bolts sheared off. The basic structure and health of our bodies is similarly affected as a result of eating poor quality foods.

Greed and dishonesty in political, business, agricultural, and medical sectors has resulted in compromised foodstuffs and medical care, with repercussions on our health. One could argue that the breakdown in the integrity and loss of discrimination in our immune system is ultimately the result of a lack of ethics, responsibility, and good values in our society.

Our cellular walls are composed of essential fatty acids, as well as cholesterol and amino acids.[22,23] Omega-3 fats regulate and normalize the proper functioning of cholesterol and Omega-6 fatty acids. When we consider that the population consuming the most fats, the Eskimos in Greenland, have little heart disease or cancer, we are led to ask, what is the difference between their diet and ours? How can they consume foods far higher in cholesterol than we do, and yet have no heart disease or cancer? One part of the answer is that Eskimos also consume plenty of Omega-3 fatty acids, which regulates how the body uses cholesterol, and we don't. Omega-3 fatty acids keep these membranes soft and fluid. When Omega-3s are absent, the other fats become hardened and the arterial walls sticky, thus, the term "hardening of the arteries."

A recent study done by the Linus Pauling Institute found that the presence of both Omega-6 fatty acids and lard caused an increase in tumor growth, whereas the presence of Omega-3 fatty acids caused a significant decrease in tumor growth.[24]

The populations of industrialized nations have built the walls of their cells from hydrogenated fats, trans fatty acids, and other poisonous fats, and now these membranes are deficient in the vital Omega-3s and other nutrients. It is becoming clear that this is a major contributor to modern disease.

# Depression

Dr. Donald Rudin and other authorities believe a deficiency of the Omega-3 fat is a main cause of depression and other mental disorders. Omega-3 fats work to keep us mentally and emotionally healthy and strong in three ways:

1. Omega-3 fats act as precursors for the body's production of key prostaglandins.
2. Omega-3 fats provide the substrate for B vitamins and co-enzymes to produce compounds that regulate many vital functions.
3. Omega-3 fats provide energy and nourishment to our nerve and brain cells.

## Eczema

One of the best-proven uses for flax seed oil and GLA is in the treatment of eczema. A malfunction in essential fatty acid metabolism has been solidly established to be a major, if not the major, cause of eczema. Many people report substantial improvement when following a nutritional program which includes 1) eliminating refined oils, excess saturated fats, and hydrogenated fats, 2) using flax seed oil and sometimes GLA, 3) taking zinc and other needed nutrients, and 4) eating a good, balanced diet.

## Fatigue

Without question, the major physical problem people have today is fatigue. We even have a disease called "Chronic Fatigue Syndrome," and while some researchers are painstakingly searching to find a viral agent as the cause of this widespread social malaise, many feel that this breakdown in people's strength and energy is caused by 1) a combination of long-standing nutritional deficiencies, and 2) an excessive intake of poisons from pharmaceuticals, drugs, our environment, and our food supply.

These two factors create conditions that lend to the development of hypothyroidism, low adrenal function, poor liver function, a weakened immune system, Candida, parasite infections, and other secondary causes of fatigue. Of these two primary causes of fatigue—nutritional deficiencies and poisons—a deficiency of the Omega-3 fats and the ingestion of considerable amounts of trans fatty acids, free radicals, and other toxic substances in refined oils are at the top of the list.

The real proof is that, people who stop using refined oils and begin including flax seed oil in their diets, report a substantial increase in energy and stamina, a softening and improvement in their skin tone, and many other positive changes.

## Heart Disease

Omega-3 fatty acids have been clearly established to lower cholesterol and triglyceride levels, and are being used extensively to both prevent and treat heart disease. Research published in 1964 in *The Lancet* showed that alpha-linolenic acid (Omega-3) and oil pressed from flax make human platelets less sticky. It has also been shown that Omega-3s lower high triglyceride levels by up to 65 percent and high cholesterol levels by up to 25 percent. Researchers recommend a tablespoonful of flax seed oil for everyone, every day, as protection against heart attack and stroke.[25]

One of the most remarkable studies on heart disease, diet, cholesterol, and refined oils is the study by Dr. Malthora presented in the *American Journal of Clinical Nutrition,* 1967, 20: 462-75. He studied a Sikh population in the north of India. They were among the world's largest consumers of clarified butter, known as "ghee." They also ate meat. While they had high serum cholesterol, they had a very low mortality rate from heart attacks.

Dr. Malthora also found a population of strict vegetarians in southern India who had almost no animal fat in their diet, but ate large amounts of refined peanut oil and margarines. These southern Indians had fifteen times as many deaths from heart attacks as the Sikhs in northern India.[26]

To further substantiate the link between refined oils and heart disease, we can examine the study of Birhard S. Rhaeja of the Jaslok Hospital in Bombay. He found that deaths from heart disease in India have greatly increased as refined vegetable oils and margarines have replaced butter and ghee in the Indian diet. The Sikhs in northern India have a much higher death rate from heart disease after including more refined oils in their diet.[27]

Other recent studies have shown that several nutrients— the Omega-3 fats, vitamin B[6], beta carotene, vitamin C, vitamin E, and chromium—have powerful antioxidant properties. They prevent free radicals from damaging cholesterol by causing it to change form and which will harden the arteries[28,29,30,31]

All of this research reveals that the real cause of heart disease is not the amount of cholesterol in the diet. Rather, it is the amount of poisons from refined oils, the lack of Omega-3 fats and a diet deficient in key antioxidants and nutrients like vitamin B[6], vitamin C, vitamin E, beta carotene, magnesium, potassium, selenium, fiber, and chromium.

Further substantiation of the realities of cholesterol and heart disease is made in the well-researched book, *The Cholesterol Conspiracy,* by Russell Smith, Ph.D., in consultation with Edward Pinckney, M.D. (Dr. Pinckney is a former associate editor of the Journal of the American Medical Association.) On the front cover of the book is a quote by George Mann, M.D., which reads, "Saturated fats and cholesterol are not the cause of coronary heart disease. That myth is the greatest scientific deception of this century, perhaps of any century."

In the Foreword, Dr. Pinckney writes, "Hitler did it. He was not the first but he did it quite successfully. 'It' being the big lie. What is even worse, the big lie about cholesterol may well kill millions of people."

The book reviews some of the common medications used to lower cholesterol. In one test with men on the drug cholestyramine, there was a 700 percent increase in colon cancer. The use of clofibrate increased total deaths by 36 percent, half of these deaths from cancer.[32]

The one limitation of the book is the authors' understanding of the dangers of consuming unsaturated fats. While they do point to tests showing an increase in cancer and other diseases from unsaturated fats, what they didn't realize is that these increases in disease are not caused by anything inherently bad about unsaturated fats, but, rather, from three other things.

1. the poisonous trans fats and free radicals created during the refining processes which are present in refined oils;

2. the absence of the antioxidant and free radical scavenging abilities of the key nutrients beta carotene, vitamin E, etc., that are removed from the oils during refining processes;

3. and the lack of Omega-3 fats in the oils they used in their tests which must be present in a ratio between one-to-one and four-to-one of Omega-6 and -3 fats for proper nourishment and good health.

We have yet to see any studies done on the use of unrefined, fresh-pressed organic vegetable oils with a proper ratio of Omega-6 and -3 fats. When these tests are done in the future, we will see that properly made vegetable oils with the right balance of essential fatty acids have quite a powerful role to play in the prevention and healing of most diseases.

On another tack, an interesting study in Finland showed that cardiac deaths were two and a half times higher in those treated with conventional medications than among those who received no medications.[33] Following is an excerpt from a different study on cardiac medications, written by Dr. Brian Leibovitz in the *Journal of Optimal Nutrition,* entitled "Nutrition: At the Crossroads."

> Drugs used for treating cardiovascular diseases are, by and large, essentially worthless (albeit these drugs are an effective means of population control). A classic example was published in the November 21, 1991 issue of NEJM (New England Journal of Medicine). This article was about a double-blind, randomized, multi-center trial of milrinone (a drug which inhibits

*phosphodiesterase*) in 1,088 patients with severe chronic heart failure.

Compared to placebo, milrinone therapy resulted in a 28 percent increase in mortality from all causes and a 34 percent increase in cardiovascular mortality.

Furthermore, milrinone significantly increased the number of serious adverse *cardiovascular* reactions and also hospitalizations as compared with the placebo group. Nice drug!

An increase in mortality after treatment with cardiac drugs is the rule, not the exception. Consider the drug clofibrate, a lipid–lowering drug prescribed for millions worldwide. In a six–year World Health Organization (WHO) study of 5,000 patients with known coronary heart disease, clofibrate–treatment resulted in a 44 percent higher mortality rate as compared to placebo.

In addition to higher mortality rates, most cardiac drugs produce a plethora of harmful side effects. Consider the drug Plendil (felodipine), a calcium channel blocker. In the latest issue of NEJM, an advertisement for Plendil lists over fifteen adverse reactions at a dose of 5 mg (in percent of patients), including: peripheral edema (22 percent), headache (19 percent), flushing (6 percent), dizziness (6 percent), upper respiratory infection (6 percent), and palpitation (2 percent). Moreover, the toxicity of Plendil is dose–dependent: at a 20 mg dose, the incidence of peripheral edema is 36 percent, palpitation 12 percent, headache 28 percent, and flushing 20 percent. The advertisement also stated that Plendil's "safety in patients with heart failure has not been established."[34]

# Immune System Viral Infections:
# Epstein Barr, Flu, HIV, and Others

Omega-3s are an essential element of many immune system processes. There has long been a great question among medical researchers and practitioners (as well as many lay people): When people are exposed to a virus, why do only a certain percentage of them become ill, while others stay healthy? For instance, in the case of Epstein Barr, a good 90 percent of the U.S. population carries this virus. Yet only a fraction will develop the illness.

Recently, some dramatic research was done which revealed important factors governing the ability of our immune systems to control and fight the ever-present pathogens to which we are exposed. Dr. David Horrobin, Dr. Stephen Wright, researchers at London Royal Free Hospital, and other scientists, have discovered evidence showing how the body's natural virus killer, interferon, is prevented from working.

Interferon is a chemical our immune system produces to kill viruses. There is now important evidence showing that the essential Omega-6 and Omega-3 fatty acids and their prostaglandin derivatives play a crucial role, both in the body's production and its utilization of interferon.

Many studies have shown that people with viral illnesses have below normal levels of the essential fatty acids and their derivatives.[35,36,37,38,39] In considering the implications of this research, Dr. Horrobin and Dr. Wright looked to the Victorian Era. At that time, children with atopic eczema became seriously ill or died after being given a smallpox vaccination, while it had no harmful effect on normal children. They theorized that these children developed eczema because they had deficiencies of essential fatty acids. This deficiency compromised their bodies' immune system and interferon's ability to fight off the smallpox virus.

To test this theory, they did a study in Ohio with first-year university students. Their essential-fatty-acid levels were tested before they went to the university. They were all found to have normal EFA levels. But after they had contracted a flu virus, they were all found to be severely deficient in the essential fatty acids.

Since then, several studies were developed to test the effectiveness of a special combination of Omega-6 fatty acids, and Omega-3 and -6 prostaglandin derivatives.

In a Scottish trial, patients with Chronic Fatigue Syndrome were given EFA supplements with great success. A double-blind, placebo-controlled trial was held for seventy patients with persistent Chronic Fatigue Syndrome, giving them linolenic acid and eicosapentaenoic acid (6-desaturated EFAs of the Omega- 6 and Omega-3 series). After six months, 84 percent of the patients in the active group, and only 22 percent of those in the placebo group, rated themselves as "better" or "much better."[40]

In another successful study, sixty-three adults with Chronic Fatigue Syndrome were enrolled in a double-blind, placebo-controlled study with essential fatty acid therapy. The patients, ill for one to three years after a viral infection, suffered from severe fatigue, myalgia, and a variety of psychological symptoms. The formula that was given contained linoleic, gamma linolenic (GLA), eicosapentaenoic (EPA), and docosahexaenoic acids (DHA). Either it or the placebo was administered over a three-month period at eight 500 mg capsules per day.

The trial was parallel in design. Patients were evaluated at entry, one month, and three months. In consultation with the patient, the doctors assessed overall condition, fatigue, myalgia, dizziness, poor concentration, and depression on a three-point scale. The essential-fatty-acid composition of their red cell membrane phospholipids was analyzed at their first and last visits.

After one month, 74 percent of patients on active treatment and 23 percent of those on placebo assessed themselves as improved over the baseline, with the improvement being much greater in the former. At three months, the corresponding figures were 85 percent and 17 percent, since the placebo group had reverted towards the baseline state, while those in the active group showed continued improvement. The essential-fatty-acid levels were abnormal at the baseline and corrected by active treatment. There were no adverse effects.[41]

The most dramatic study to date has been one on AIDS patients at the Muhimbili Medical Center at the University of Dar Es Salaam, Tanzania. In that country, only 7.5 percent of AIDS patients live longer than three months. Treatment with the essential fatty acid blend resulted in substantial improvement in health in all thirteen patients participating in the study.

Patients were treated with a special blend of the essential fatty acids—gamma linolenic acid (GLA), eicosapentaenoic acid (EPA), and docosahexaenoic acid (DHA). They experienced weight gain; a rise in CD4 lymphocyte levels; reduction in fatigue, diarrhea, and skin rashes; and improved survival. Two patients improved so much they were able to return to work. Twenty months later, five are still alive and "relatively well."[42]

An excellent summary regarding EFAs and viral infections was presented by Dr. Horrobin of the Efamol Research Institute in an article called "Post-Viral Fatigue Syndrome, Viral Infections in Atopic Eczema, and Essential Fatty Acids."

> There are several interesting interrelationships between EFA metabolism and viral infections.
>
> **1. EFAs have direct antiviral** effects and are lethal at surprisingly low concentrations to many viruses, notably those which have a lipid envelope. The antiviral activity of human milk seems to be largely attributable to its EFA content.
>
> **2. Interferons cannot exert any antiviral effects in cells in which the cyclo-oxygenase enzyme is either blocked or absent.** This presumably means that interferon requires one or other cyclo-oxygenase metabolites to exert its effect. Interferon is an effective stimulator of the cyclo-oxygenase and many of its side effects relate to formation of

cyclo-oxygenase metabolites. If interferon requires the enzyme in order to exert its antiviral actions, then substrate for that enzyme must also be available. Thus, in the absence of adequate EFA substrate concentrations, the efficacy of interferon will be reduced.

**3. Several different viruses which infect mammalian cells in vitro are able to inhibit the enzyme 6-desaturase.** Inhibition of 6-desaturation is likely to be an effective strategy for a virus attacking a cell. Blockade of 6-desaturation will render the cell unable to make the substrates such as DGLA, AA, and EPA, required for the cyclo-oxygenase. This will thus lead to reduced antiviral efficacy of interferon. In evolutionary terms, inhibition of 6-desaturation would be a highly advantageous characteristic for a virus to acquire.

**4. Viral infections lower blood levels of EFAs.** This was first observed over recently, it has been confirmed in the case of EB virus infections. There was prolonged lowering of blood EFA levels lasting at least several months. The details of the EFA pattern indicated inhibition of EFA desaturation with little effect on elongation as would be expected from the known in vitro actions of viruses. Of particular interest was the observation that at eight and twelve months those who had recovered clinically showed normal or near-normal EFA blood levels. In contrast, those who were still clinically ill showed persistently abnormal EFA levels. Similar but much more severe reductions in blood EFA concentrations have recently been demonstrated in patients with acquired immune deficiency syndrome.[43]

This by no means infers that the use of essential fatty acids is a cure for AIDS and other viral illnesses, or even the sole or primary cause. It certainly seems clear, however, that considering all the information and research presented in this book and elsewhere, it is reasonable to state that essential fatty acids play a key role in a healthy, functioning immune system. When they are deficient, the immune system will be weakened. Careful use of balanced amounts of essential fatty acids and, in some cases, their prostaglandin derivatives, is an important part of a nutritional program.

## Metabolism

EFAs increase cellular metabolic rate, thereby increasing energy and stamina.

## Pain and Inflammation

Pain and inflammation are controlled in certain ways by the prostaglandins 1 and 3 series, derived from the Omega-3 and Omega-6 fatty acids. The prostaglandins 2 series, on the other hand, increases pain and inflammation from injuries. It is derived from arachidonic acid, which is present in meat, thus if the body is lacking the fats and prostaglandins that control pain and inflammation while having an excess of the other fats and prostaglandins that increase pain, an unnecessary and painful reaction to injury or other stimuli may occur—one that could have been controlled or even eliminated by a healthy body's normal processes.

When we study the research, we discover that the essential fats relieve rheumatoid arthritis, PMS, depression, heart disease, cancer and even more recently, Chronic Fatigue Syndrome, and AIDS. We can't help but wonder, if these fats cause such relief of these illnesses, then is a serious deficiency of these fats partially responsible for causing them?

## PMS

One of the most thoroughly tested uses of Omega-3 fatty acids and GLA has been to help alleviate the symptoms of PMS.[44,45] A woman's menstrual cycle is regulated mainly by her female hormones (estrogen and progesterone), as well as thyroid hormones, vitamins (especially B6), minerals, and prostaglandins. PMS is usually caused by a deficiency or imbalance in the estrogen and progesterone hormones and prostaglandins.

The Omega-6 and Omega-3 essential fatty acids are precursors (raw materials) from which the prostaglandins are made. Any deficiency or imbalance in the Omega-6 and -3 fats will create a corresponding disorder in the prostaglandins, which can contribute to PMS symptoms. Some women are unable to properly convert the Omega-6 fat into GLA, which is then converted into prostaglandins. These women often benefit greatly from taking a GLA supplement in the form of borage seed oil or evening primrose oil, along with using flax seed oil daily.[46] Eliminating the wrong fats from one's diet, eating well, and taking additional supplements like vitamin E, Beauty Pearls (a Chinese herbal formula), and a low potency B complex formula, preferably from Food Form Vitamins, also helps.

## Prostaglandins

One of the most important functions of Omega-3s and Omega-6s is to provide the raw material for the body to manufacture prostaglandins, the hormonelike compounds that regulate many bodily functions.

## Skin conditions

Eczema, dry skin, and other skin conditions are often caused by a deficiency of Omega-3 fatty acids. Many people have found that regular use of flax seed oil has greatly improved their skin condition.

## Ulcers

Ulcers are one of the most widespread illnesses afflicting modern man today. As a matter of fact, the foremost selling pharmaceutical is an antacid formula. No doubt poor diet, the stresses of urban living, and dehumanized and disempowering working conditions all contribute their share to this condition.

Interestingly, it has been discovered that the prostaglandins series plays a part in both regulating the amount of stomach acid produced, and in maintaining a strong, healthy digestive tract lining. Dr. Charles Bates, in his noteworthy book, *Essential Fatty Acids in Health and Disease,* describes the recoveries of many of his patients from digestive disorders following the use of essential fatty acids and GLA.

## Other Conditions

Other conditions that have been helped by EFAs include dry eyes, psoriasis, diabetes, multiple sclerosis, schizophrenia, and nervous system dysfunctions.

1.  Charles Bates, Ph.D., *Essential Fatty Acids and Immunity in Mental Health* (Washington: Life Sciences Press, 1987).
2.  Donald O. Rudin, M.D., *The Omega-3 Phenomenon* (New York: Rawson Associates, 1987).
3.  Judy Graham, *Evening Primrose Oil* (New York: Thorsons, 1984).

4. Ibid.
5. Ibid.
6. John Finnegan, and Daphne Gray, *Recovery from Addiction* (Berkeley: Celestial Arts, 1990).
7. Robert B. Gennis, *Biomembranes Molecular Structure and Function* (New York: Springer-Verlag, 1989).
8. Bates, op. cit.
9. Bruce Alberts, et al., *Molecular Biology of the Cell* (New York: Garland Publishing, 1989).
10. Bates, op. cit.
11. Udo Erasmus, *Fats and Oils* (Canada: Alive, 1986).
12. Udo Erasmus, *Fats That Heal, Fats That Kill* Designing Health (1988): 18.
13. *JNCI*, Vol. 77, No. 5 (Nov. 1986): 1053–1061.
14. Dr. Johanna Budwig, *Flax Oil As A True Aid Against Arthritis, Heart Infarction, Cancer and Other Diseases* (Vancouver, Canada: Apple Publishing, 1992).
15. Erasmus, *Fats and Oils*, op. cit.
16. Ibid.
17. *JAOCS*, Vol. 65, No. 4 (April 1988): 509 (summary).
18. The Linus Pauling Institute of Science and Medicine, Palo Alto, California.
19. Erasmus, *Fats and Oils*, op. cit.
20. Gennis, op. cit.
21. Alberts, et al., op. cit.
22. Gennis, op. cit.
23. Alberts, et al., op. cit.
24. The Linus Pauling Institute, op. cit.
25. *The Lancet*, Vol. 2 (July–December 1964): 975–979.
26. Dr. Malthora, *American Journal of Clinical Nutrition*, 20 (1967): 462–475.
27. Birhard S. Rhaeja, *The Lancet* (November 14, 1987).
28. W.J. Serfontein, et al., "Plasma Pyridoxal-5-Phosphate Level as Risk Index for Coronary Artery Disease," *Atherosclerosis* 55 (1985): 357–61.
29. "Is Vitamin B6 an Antithrombotic Agent?" *The Lancet* 1 (1981): 1299–1300.
30. J.F. Rhinehart, and L.D. Greenberg, "Vitamin B6 Deficiency in the Rhesus Monkey, with Particular Reference to the Occurrence of Atherosclerosis, Dental Caries and Hepatic Cirrhosis," *American Journal of Clinical Nutrition* 4 (1956): 318.
31. E. Bendit, "The Origin of Atherosclerosis," *Scientific American*, 236–2 (February 1977): 74–85.
32. Russell L. Smith, Ph.D. with Edward R. Pinckney, M.D., *The Cholesterol Conspiracy* (St. Louis: Warren H. Green, Inc., 1991).
33. T.E. Strandberg, et al., *JAMA*, 266:1225–1229.
34. Brian Leibovitz, Ph.D., "Nutrition: At The Crossroads," *Journal of Optimal Nutrition*, Vol 1, Number 1 (1992).
35. Peter O. Behan, and Wilhelmina M.H. Behan, "Essential Fatty Acids in the Treatment of Postviral Fatigue Sydrome," *Omega-6 Fatty Acids, Pathophysiology and Roles in Clinical Medicine* (Alan R. Liss, Inc.: 1990): 275–282.
36. P.O. Behan, W.M.H. Behan, and D. Horrobin, "Effect of high doses of essential fatty acids on the postviral fatigue syndrome," *Acta Neurol Scand* 82 (1990): 209–216.
37. Lowell L. Williams, et al., "Serum Fatty Acid Proportions Are Altered During the Year Following Acute Epstein-Barr Virus Infection," *Lipids*, Vol. 23, No. 10 (1988).
38. D.F. Horrobin, "Post-Viral Fatigue Sydrome, Viral Infections in Atopic Eczema, and Essential Fatty Acids," *Medical Hypotheses*, 32 (1990): 211–217.
39. K. Palangyo, et al., "An Open Study of Essential Fatty Acid Therapy (Efamol Marine) in Patients with AIDS," (a study, available from Efamol).
40. Behan, Peter O., et al., op. cit.
41. Behan, P.O., et al., op. cit.
42. Palangyo, K., et al., op. cit.
43. Horrobin, D.F., op. cit.
44. Rudin, op. cit.
45. Bates, op. cit.
46. Graham, op. cit.

# CHAPTER 11

# Weight Management: A Balanced Approach

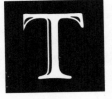his may come as a great surprise, but eating fat (the right kind of fat) can help you lose weight. Overwhelming evidence shows that the Omega-3 and Omega-6 essential fatty acids stimulate the body's burning of "brown" fat. They also act as solvents to help the body dissolve and remove hard fats.

Overweight people in today's modern society are quite often starving for fat—a certain kind of fat. Because eating habits have changed so dramatically in the past century, our bodies are deficient in the Omega-3 essential fatty acid, while they contain excessive amounts of the harmful hydrogenated fats, trans fatty acids, and saturated fats. Some medical studies show that our diets today have only from one-sixteenth to one-twentieth the amount of Omega-3 fats that they contained a hundred years ago. At the same time, we are eating twenty to one hundred times as much hydrogenated fats and trans fatty acids.

Many of my friends and clients report that, after adding

one to two tablespoons a day of flax seed oil to their diets and eliminating poisonous fats, they have lost cravings for fatty foods and have experienced continued weight loss, increased energy, and a sense of dietary satisfaction.

When the body is deficient in the Omega-3 fatty acids, it continuously sends a message to the brain, saying, "FAT! I NEED FATS!" Because most of us can't distinguish between the various types of fats, and until recently, the right kinds of fats were not even available, we head straight for the ice cream, pies, margarines, butter, salad dressings, french fries, and other fatty foods to satiate our cravings for fat. Unfortunately, we only exacerbate the problem because the more we consume the wrong kind of fats, the greater the imbalance and deficiency of the right kind of fats becomes.

It is amazing to think that in a land of so many overweight people, where such high levels of fat are consumed, most of us are literally starving for fat, the Omega-3 essential fatty acid. Furthermore, nearly all of the major diseases today in Western nations—from heart disease and cancer, to arthritis, fatigue, PMS, and immune system weakness—are partially caused by a deficiency of the essential fatty acids, especially the Omega-3s.

There are five main physical factors involved in weight management, whether one is concerned with being underweight or overweight. They are:

1. **Metabolism**
2. **Diet**
3. **Nutrition**
4. **Exercise**
5. **Disease**

A malfunctioning metabolism is often the main cause of the overweight or underweight condition. However, it can be corrected through proper diet, nutrition, exercise, and the healing of any diseases that influence weight. We all know people who can eat as much as they want without gaining weight, so likewise, it must be true that a metabolism disorder often underlies excessive weight gain.

Although starvation-thin figures are the rage among to-day's models, a modicum of fat is beneficial, as it provides extra fuel during times of hard work, travel, and other stressful occasions when it may be difficult to eat well. A little extra fat on our figures also helps to keep blood sugar stable, provides warmth, and insulates our organs from injury. However, being seriously overweight can damage one's health and contribute to many serious diseases and conditions including:

> Heart Disease, High Cholesterol, High Blood Pressure, Hypothyroidism, Arthritis, Cancer, Diabetes, Constipation, Varicose Veins, Anorexia, Bulimia, Candida, Cellulite, Fatigue, and PMS.

Many people have found that a good nutrition and exercise program that enables them to lose excess weight will also create a substantial increase in energy, and alleviate associated health problems.

Popular diets often recommend eliminating all fats to lose weight. While limiting some fats is highly recommended, eliminating all fats can lead to nutritional deficiencies and serious health problems. Millions upon millions of people—especially women—are unknowingly causing severe damage to their health from poorly conceived weight-loss programs that eliminate key fats from the diet. Millions of unborn children will be condemned to a lifetime of suffering from maldeveloped brain, immune, and nervous systems caused by their mother's dietary deficiency of the Omega-3 fatty acid and the toxic effects of trans fatty acids, free radicals, and other poisonous substances in their consumption of refined oils.

Fats that should be eliminated from the diet are the chemically altered fats found in commercial margarines, shortenings, cooking and salad oils, and processed foods. The harmful effects of these oils have been described in chapters 3 and 10. Decreasing the amount of animal fats is also important. Choose lean cuts of meat, remove the skin from chicken, and include fish in the diet, particularly poached or baked salmon, tuna, trout, and others high in the Omega-3 and Omega-6 essential fatty acids. These EFAs help to properly metabolize other fats and prevent the buildup of plaque in the arteries.

## Flax Seed Oil: A Dieter's Dream

Although some EFAs can be obtained from fish, the best source is unrefined vegetable oil. Canola oil, pumpkin seed oil, soybean oil, and walnut oil all contain both Omega-3 and Omega-6 essential fatty acids. However, fresh flax seed oil contains the highest amounts of Omega-3 fats and is the best source of these fats.

It has been found that mixing flax seed oil with protein is a winning combination with regard to both health and weight management. Animal tests showed that a diet high in protein without EFAs caused severe deficiencies and obesity. When EFAs were added to their diet, health and normal weight were restored.[1] Many doctors recommend a combination of low-fat cottage cheese and flax seed oil in the treatment of patients suffering from a wide array of maladies, from cancer to obesity.

The diet recommended here includes the following foods: whole grains and beans, a wide variety of fresh vegetables (both raw and cooked), fish, chicken and fowl, lean meats, eggs, low-fat dairy products (in moderation), whole grain breads, and some fresh fruit. Low-fat cottage cheese, mixed with a tablespoon of fresh flax seed oil, should be taken once or twice daily. Only high quality, certified organic, unrefined, fresh-pressed oils made by a reputable company like Omega Nutrition and Arrowhead Mills should be used for dressings and sauces. As much as is practical, all foods should be fresh, certified organic, and properly prepared so as to avoid the loss of vital nutrients.

Foods to avoid include: saturated fats, processed foods, simple carbohydrates (pastries, refined breads and flour products, refined sugars), chemically altered fats (margarines, shortenings, fried foods), sugar, and caffeine. One should also avoid alcoholic beverages, smoking, recreational drugs, cakes, candies, and ice cream. Also recommended is one to two tablespoons daily of cold-pressed, organic flax seed oil, to meet the necessary quota of the essential Omega-3 and Omega-6 fatty acids.

## Weight Management and Nutritional Formulas

Some people will find their weight will normalize just from a good diet, the right oils, and exercise. Others who have a malfunctioning metabolism, either because of genetic inheritance or from damage to their health through years of poor nutrition, illness, and / or drug abuse, will need additional support from extra vitamin, mineral, and herbal formulas to restore their health and their bodies' fat metabolism processes.

However, be wary. There are many programs that cause serious damage to people's health, programs that reduce their muscle content, create nutritional deficiencies, and have a "rebound effect," where dieters end up regaining more fat and having less muscle mass than they had previously. This occurs because many of these programs don't provide complete nutrition with a balanced understanding and use of properly made oils.

There are a few good nutritional formulas on the market that help reduce excess weight in a beneficial way. These formulas provide people with essential nutrients they are lacking, and assist their overall health and fat-burning functions. People also find that their energy increases substantially using these formulas. When combined with a balanced diet and the right oils, they can be quite helpful.

The formulas are produced by Lifephase, Omega Nutrition, Metagenics / Ethical Nutrients, Sunrider International, and other companies. They are available from natural foods stores, health practitioners, and independent distributors. (The phone numbers and addresses of these companies are listed in this book under Sources of Products.) Some recommended herbal and nutritional formulas are:

> Acidophilus, Action Caps, Aloe Vera, Apple cider
> vinegar, Beauty Pearls, Calli tea, Chromium

Piccolinate, Flax seed meal, Flax seed oil, Fortune Delight tea, Nuplus, Prime Again, Slimphase #1 and #2, Stevia, SunBar, UltraBalance, and UltraClear.

## Weight Management Program:

Make a tea combining 1–2 bags of Calli tea with 1–2 small packs of Fortune Delight in 2 quarts of water. Add your favorite herbal sweetener and drink all day.

Take 2 to 3 tablets of Slimphase #1 with breakfast and lunch and take 10 to 15 drops of Slimphase #2 under the tongue three times a day.

Take 1 tsp. to 1 Tbs. apple cider vinegar one to three times a day in 4 oz. warm water with meals.

Use the Action Caps and other formulas as well.

Use the UltraClear or UltraBalance, and NuPlus formulas by themselves or in smoothies. Blend them with flax seed oil and flax seed meal or Nutri-Flax.

## Smoothie Recipe:

Here is a suggested smoothie recipe that combines many key nutrients and tastes great. Try your own variations with your favorite ingredients. Drink once or twice a day instead of meals.

Make the smoothies in a base of Calli and/or Fortune Delight tea and add Chinese herbal formulas as desired:

12–16 oz. water, Calli/Fortune Delight tea and/or fruit juice
3–4 squirts Stevia sweetener
1–3 Tbs. NuPlus
1–2 scoops UltraClear or UltraBalance
1–3 Tbs. Nutri-Flax
1–2 tsp. flax seed oil
1 tsp. or 1–2 tablets acidophilus
add fruit and/or yogurt if desired

For a more effective, complete program, take the following supplements with it:

2–3 Slimphase tablets
6–9 Action Caps
1 Beauty Pearl
2 Prime Again
1 Chromium Piccolinate
1–3 tsp. apple cider vinegar (mixed in water)
½–1 oz. aloe vera concentrate (in 4 oz. water)

**Note:** Take aloe vera concentrate a half hour before each smoothie and each meal. The aloe vera will help to normalize digestive secretions, increase metabolism, and kill pathogenic bacteria, parasites, and yeast.

People who would like further information on good nutrition, with additional recipes, are referred to *The Facts About Fats Cookbook* by John Finnegan and Kathy Cituk, and *Weight Management: A Balanced Approach* by John Finnegan and Kathy Cituk, published by Elysian Arts Press. People who would like additional help with sugar, caffeine, and other addictions will find excellent guidance in the book *Recovery From Addiction* by John Finnegan and Daphne Gray, published by Celestial Arts.

Most aloe drinks on the market have very few active ingredients. To obtain results it is essential to use a real brand like AloeNique or R PUR Aloe that have been proven to contain high amounts of the active ingredients.

> ❧

1.  William L. Fischer, *How to Fight Cancer and Win* (Canada: Alive, 1987).

# CHAPTER 12

# The Vital Role of Essential Fatty Acids for Pregnant and Nursing Women

R ecently it has been discovered that the Omega-3 fats are necessary for the complete development of the human brain during pregnancy and the first two years of life. The Omega-3 fat and its derivative, DHA (docosahexaenoic acid), is so essential to a child's development that if a mother and infant are deficient in it, the child's nervous system and immune system may never fully develop, and it can cause a lifetime of unexplained emotional, learning, and immune system disorders.

Considering the enormous increase in emotional, learning, and immune system disorders in our population today, one can't help but wonder what effect this widespread nutritional deficiency is having on the breakdown today in people's health.

One also wonders whether the prevalence of infant and childhood illnesses like diaper rash; Epstein Barr; Candida albicans overgrowth; sinus allergies; chronic ear, nose, and throat infections; as well as so-called emotional disorders like hyper-activity and autistic behavior also have their basis in nutritional deficiencies, particularly in the lack of Omega-3 fatty acids.

Further compounding the problem, an estimated 60-70 percent of all two-month-old babies are bottle-fed, and 75-80 percent of all four-month-old babies are bottle-fed; none of the powdered baby formulas such as Isomil, Similac, Gerber, and Carnation contain Omega-3 fatty acids.[1] To my knowledge, all baby formulas are made with commercially processed oils which contain high levels of poisonous trans fatty acids and other harmful compounds.[2]

Dr. Donald Rudin, in his excellent book *The Omega-3 Phenomenon,* states the issue succinctly:

> There is no comparable substitute for the remarkable mix of nutrients and immunity-boosting factors provided by mother's milk, as long as the mother is eating properly. A well-nourished nursing mother provides her infant with a perfect blend of essential fatty acids and their long-chained derivatives, assuring the fast-growing brain and body tissues a rich sup-ply. Mother's milk also supplies important anti-bodies not present in cow's milk or in artificial formula. Here is a nutritive comparison:
>
> • Breast milk may have five times more arachidonic acid and two and a half times more EPA (eicosapentaenoic acid) than formula.
> • Breast milk may have thirty times more DHA (docosahexaenoic acid) than formula.
> • Compared with mother's milk, formu-las are also low in selenium and biotin.
>
> Sadly, the breast milk of many mothers in our country reflects the high trans fatty acid

and low Omega-3 content in the average diet.
American mothers produce milk that often has
only one-fifth to one-tenth of the Omega-3
content of the milk that well-nourished, nut-
eating Nigerian mothers provide their infants.

This discovery has far-reaching implications. A study in March,
1991 at the Mayo Clinic of nineteen "normal" pregnant women
consuming normal diets indicated all were deficient in the
Omega-3 fats and to a lesser degree, Omega-6 fats.[3] Another
study of Inuit (Eskimo) women, compared to Canadian women,
revealed the same deficiencies in the milk of Canadian nursing
mothers.[4]

Compounding the problem is our nation's pervasive ob-
session with weight loss programs, which induce women to
avoid all fats. The frightening news is that for the past three
generations (since the advent of refined oils), the vast majority
of the population in North America has not been given adequate nourishment for complete brain development. The part
of the brain that Omega-3 effects is the learning ability, anxiety /
depression, and auditory and visual perception. The Omega-3
fats also aid in balancing the autoimmune system, and there
seem to be a growing number of children with allergies, colic,
and skin problems.

There are also indications that Omega-3 fats play an ongoing role in brain function, healthy immune system function,
and general growth throughout childhood and adolescence. One
study revealed that Omega-3 supplementation induced catch-up
growth in a deficient, underdeveloped seven-year-old.[5]

Since our mental apparatus is developed in the mother's
womb and during the first two years of life, one would be wise
to heed the advice of the researchers from the Mayo Clinic
study.[6] They suggest that this important fat be supplemented
in every pregnancy, and that refined and hydrogenated fats be
avoided during this critical period.

For these conservative researchers to include a message
like this in their research paper should make us concerned for our

future. I have personal experience with families who have had flax babies. These children (now 3 and 6 years old) are very bright and healthy and have been free from many health problems most young children now experience.

A deficiency of the Omega-3 and Omega-6 fats causes insufficient milk production and breast engorgement. Flax seed oil has been found to substantially increase milk production in women who are not producing enough milk to nurse their infants. It also often clears up breast engorgement. One woman I know was having great difficulty producing enough milk to nurse her newborn child. Within twenty-four hours of taking flax seed oil, her milk production doubled, and one breast that was engorged opened up, allowing the milk to flow freely.

Many authorities recommend that pregnant and nursing women consume fatty fish two to three times weekly and/or add a minimal amount of flax seed oil to their diets to insure adequate intake of Omega-6 and Omega-3 fatty acids.

Another paper worth reading is the report given by Artemis Simopoulos, M.D., a pediatrician and endocrinologist from the International Life Sciences Institute.[7] She takes a comprehensive look at how the Omega-3 deficiency affects many areas, from fetal growth to arthritis and cancer.

A healthy mother's milk is high in essential fatty acids, GLA, and other precursors to prostaglandins. Cow's milk is low in essential fatty acids, and other prostaglandin precursors, and is high in saturated fats. For this reason, cow's milk is not an adequate substitute for mother's milk. Neither is baby formula. At a recent international symposium on "Dietary Omega-3 and -6 Fatty Acids," Dr. Neuringer, an authority on infant milk, stated that the low Omega-3, high Omega-6 content in infant formulas is of great concern because of the imbalance it causes among the resultant prostaglandins. These imbalances could impair the immune system and predispose the infant to cancer and heart trouble later in life. Feeding a nonnursing baby a few drops of flax seed oil will provide the Omega-3 and Omega-6 essential fatty acids.

The Health Protection Branch of the Canadian government, which is the equivalent of the American FDA, is considering requiring that all infant formulas contain adequate amounts of the Omega-3 fatty acids.

Flax seed oil is the highest source of Omega-3 fatty acids, a good source of the Omega-6 fatty acids, and has no cholesterol. It is good tasting and can be poured directly onto protein dishes, vegetables, salads, grains, and soups. It is a very delicate oil and should not be used for cooking.

Authorities recommend that 2 percent of daily calories be composed of Omega-3 fatty acids, which can be provided by the following amounts of flax seed oil:

¼ teaspoon for nonnursing infants 1 to 6 months
½ teaspoon for nonnursing infants 6 to 12 months
1–2 teaspoons for 1- to 2-year-olds
2 teaspoons for children over 2 years
1–2 tablespoons for adults

**Note:** Since most adults today are deficient in the Omega-3 fatty acids, nursing mothers may not have sufficient amounts to pass along to their infants. It is especially important, therefore, for pregnant and nursing women to supplement their diets with flax seed oil. A few drops can be added to infant formulas and rubbed on the infant's abdomen.

## Generational Consequences of Deficiency

There are many serious consequences of generation after generation having diets deficient in an element essential for normal development of the nervous system. Following are a few observations of the effects that inadequate nutrition is having on social and economic conditions today.

- A widespread alienation and pervasive depression in young people, truly alarming to observe in an age group usually known for its boundless enthusiasm and enjoyment of life.
- An increase in suicides and killings among

young children, almost unheard of a generation ago.

• The ongoing increase in drug and alcohol abuse.
• An unparalleled growth of immune system disorders like Epstein Barr, Candida, allergies, chronic sinus and ear infections, and digestive disorders.
• A serious decline in the level of scholastic achievement amongst school children.
• A continued deterioration of the quality of goods produced by American industries. (A nation of people that lives on hamburgers, french fries, milk shakes, cola drinks, TV dinners, and other toxic foods is destined to lose its competitive edge, and will continue to foster drug abuse in the workplace.)

Certainly, there are many social and economic factors contributing to this disturbing state of the health of our people. But there is also a great deal of sound scientific research that clearly demonstrates that, when populations are subjected to serious, continued nutritional deficiencies, the offspring of each successive generation shows an increased deterioration in physical and mental health.[8,9,10,11,12,13] I have spoken with many older doctors who have told me that they find most people in their fifties and sixties to be constitutionally stronger and healthier than those of the next generation, in their thirties and forties.

In his classic work, *Nutrition and Physical Degeneration,* Dr. Weston Price presents remarkable observations on the diets and health of different cultures around the world. He has extensively documented the degeneration that occurs when healthy peoples, eating traditional diets, convert to modern foods.

Dr. Price's time in history was unique. He was able to observe many cultures, living and eating as they had for thousands of years. When these people met the modern age and converted to modern diets, they experienced disastrous consequences to their physical and emotional health.

He studied society after society, from Swiss farmers living in high Alpine valleys to Gaelics on islands of the outer Hebrides, from descendants of ancient civilizations living in Peru to the Maori in New Zealand, the Eskimos in Alaska, Indians in Canada and the United States, Melanesians and Polynesians in the South Pacific, Africans and Malay tribes on islands north of Australia. Again and again, he found the same story repeated. The indigenous peoples had strong, healthy bodies, free from cancer, heart disease, and immune system weakness. And surprisingly, tooth decay and cavities were almost nonexistent, despite the fact that these peoples usually had no dentists or fluoride toothpaste. Nor did they fluoridate their water supplies.[14,15]

He saw, firsthand, how each succeeding generation that converted their diets to modern, refined foods experienced a continued deterioration in health. He also met several doctors who told him that, in several decades of living among native peoples, they never saw a single case of cancer.

❧

1.  C. CF Liu, et al. "Increase in plasma phasonalipid DHA and EFAs as a reflection of their intake and mode of administration," *Pediatr. Res.* 22 (1987): 292–6.
2.  Bonnie Liebman, "Baby Formula: Missing Key Fats?" *Nutrition Action Healthletter* (October 1990): 8–9.
3.  Ralph T. Holman, Susan Johnson, Paul Ogburn, "Deficiency of essential fatty acids and membrane fluidity during pregnancy and lactation," *Biochemistry,* Proc. Natl. Acad. Sci. USA, Vol. 88 (June 1991): 4835–4839.
4.  Sheila M. Innis, and Harriet V. Kuhnlein, "Long-chain n-3 fatty acids in breast milk of Inuit women consuming traditional foods," *Early Human Development* 18 (Elsevier Scientific Publishers Ireland Ltd.: 1988): 185–189.
5.  Bjerve K.S., Thoereson, "Linseed oil and cod liver oil induce rapid growth in a seven-year-old girl with a N-3 fatty acid deficient," JPEN, *J. Parenter, Enteral Nutr.* 12(5) (Sept.– Oct. 1988): 521–5.
6.  Ralph Holman, et al., op. cit.
7.  Artemis Simopoulos, M.D., *Nutrition Today,* March/April 1988 & May/June 1988.
8.  Weston Price, *Nutrition and Physical Degeneration* (La Mesa, California: Price-Pottenger Nutrition Foundation, 1954).
9.  Elaine Pottenger, and Robert Pottenger, Jr., eds. *Pottenger's Cats: A Study in Nutrition* (edited writings of Francis Pottenger) (La Mesa, California: The Price-Pottenger Nutrition Foundation, 1983).
10. Alexander G. Schauss, M.D., *Crime, Diet & Delinquency* (California: Parker House, 1981).
11. Bernard Jensen and Mark Anderson, *Empty Harvest* (New York: Avery, 1990).
12. Dr. Johanna Budwig, *Flax Oil as a True Aid against Arthritis, Heart Infarction, Cancer and Other Diseases* (Vancouver, Canada: Apple Publishing, 1992).
13. Ronald F. Schmid, M.D., *Traditional Foods Are Your Best Medicine* (New York: Ballantine, 1987).
14. Price, op. cit.
15. Schmid, op. cit.

# CHAPTER 13

# Essential Fatty Acids for Fitness and Athletic Performance

R ecently, one of the nation's most famous football stars died from a brain tumor that he claimed to be the result of from his use of steroids. The media continues to bring us alarming stories about the widespread and dangerous use of steroids among athletes and fitness buffs. Even high school students have succumbed to the illusory pursuit of fame and glory at the inestimable cost of their health.

What is continually overlooked are the simple but powerful methods to build up strength and muscle tissue that nature offers through the use of good, wholesome organic foods; Chinese tonic herbal formulas; superfoods like bee pollen; vitamin and mineral formulas; flax seed oil; and the flax seed oil–protein combination.

Athletes, body builders, and fitness buffs often use a high carbohydrate, high protein, low fat diet. This is limited according to many studies. The optimal diet for building strength and energy is composed of a balanced amount of carbohydrates, proteins, Omega-3 and Omega-6 essential fatty acids, vitamins, and minerals.

Many athletes report that by adding one or two table-spoons of flax seed oil a day to a high-powered smoothie drink, or by putting it on food, they achieve their best performance. A man I know in his sixties, chairman of the board of a major corporation, wrote, "I climbed the highest peak in the Rockies, traversing over twenty miles with an altitude gain and descent of over five thousand feet without tiring after months of using a tablespoon or so per day of flax seed oil, and I feel that the extra oxygenation in my blood was a direct result. A year before, I had climbed a lesser peak with more difficulty."

Many athletes also find a substantially increased perfor-mance level with the oxygen- and energy-carrying functions of flax seed oil and the lipoprotein combination, which creates a synergistic effect. (The oil-protein formulas are discussed in chapter 9.)

ed.

# CHAPTER 14

# How Much Oil to Use?

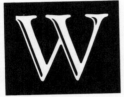e know we have to change something when more than three-quarters of the population are dying from heart disease, cancer, and other diseases that scarcely existed a hundred years ago. It is obvious that we are doing something wrong. It is difficult to find a clear answer because there has been such a thorough breakdown in our social structure and the radical change in the production and preparation of our foods has obscured the memory of our cultural heritage.

I personally have sought an answer to this question from four sources. The first is my own personal experience—seeing what nourishes and heals me. The second is listening to my friends and clients; the third, objectively examining hard-core scientific research; and the fourth, looking at the studies of societies of people who live long, healthy lives, free of most diseases.

In looking at the diet and nutrition of traditional, healthy peoples, some answers came to light. First, there are no records of healthy societies where people lived exclusively on brown rice and vegetables, carrot juice, wheatgrass juice, or sprouts; nor, for that matter, did they consume hot dogs, french fries, milk shakes, ice cream, TV dinners, soft drinks filled with caffeine, sugar or artificial sweeteners, or other such creations of the modern chemical laboratories. While there have been a few healthy vegetarian cultures, most of them have not been strictly vegetarian. Instead, their diets have had a broader base, using dairy products, eggs, fish, fowl, and some, meat.[1,2]

Healthy cultures were well-nourished, with most eating plenty of vegetables, some fruit, some grains or a form of tuber, and nearly all having good sources of high quality fat and protein in the form of beans, seafood, dairy foods, wild game, or free-range fowl and livestock. It is important to note that all their food was either from wild sources or organically grown.[3]

What no healthy society had in their diet were caged animals (as opposed to free-range or wild); processed oils, refined sugar, refined and bleached flour products; synthetic preservatives and food colorings; pesticides and herbicides; synthetic, acidulated fertilizers; chlorine in the water supply; or a host of other poisonous compounds that exist today in our food, air, and water. The other common denominator of healthy peoples is that they did a great deal of physical work—fishing, farming, hunting, building, washing, cooking, and walking.

One thing that becomes clear when one studies these cultures is that, while there are general guidelines, there is also a great deal of individual variation or, "biochemical individuality." Some peoples have a much higher or different metabolism than others, do more vigorous physical work, or have a more active lifestyle, and their bodies need several times as much fat as others do. Others, through genetic heritage or illness, may tolerate only small amounts of very high quality oils in their diets.

As a general guideline, most people need anywhere from 15-30 percent of their calories from a combination of saturated and unsaturated fats, which is two-and-one-half to five tablespoons per day. This includes salad oils, cooking oils, and fats in foods including beans, nuts and seeds, meat, fish, and poultry. Of this amount, at least half should be Omega-6 fatty acids and one-half to one-fourth should be Omega-3 fatty acids.[4,5]

A study by Dr. Artemis Simopoulos determined that our ancestors traditionally ate diets with a one-to-one ratio of Omega-6 and Omega-3 fats.[6] In practical terms, this means about two tablespoons of sunflower or a similar type of oil, and one to two tablespoons of flax seed oil; or two to three table-spoons per day of Essential Balance (a special blend of flax seed and sunflower seed oil), giving a one-to-one ratio of Omega-6s to Omega-3s. That, combined with some olive or hazelnut oil or butter, will yield the minimum daily requirements for essential and nonessential fatty acids. Some people will function optimally on substantially higher amounts of fats, although they should be good quality, unprocessed oils. People need to develop an awareness of their own body's needs.

People with heart disease, cancer, or similar illnesses can use a larger amount of flax seed oil—one to two tablespoons or more—for the first few months, until their Omega-3 deficiency is restored to normal. Some people believe that when a large amount of flax oil is taken, 400 iu (international units) or more of vitamin E should also be taken. These illnesses are partially caused by a lifetime of poor dietary habits, and consuming excessive amounts of saturated, hydrogenated and trans fats. They need to be very careful to eliminate all forms of saturated and trans fats and all processed oils from their diet.

There are five changes in fat consumption in the average Western diet that must be made in order to eliminate the toxins from fats, correct deficiencies and imbalances, and restore health. These are:

1. Reduce overall fat intake.
2. Eliminate processed oils from diet.
3. Reduce saturated fat intake.
4. Use correct amount of the Omega-3 fatty acids.
5. Use correct amount of the Omega-6 fatty acids.

1. Ronald Schmid, *Traditional Foods Are Your Best Medicine* (New York: Ballantine, 1987).
2. Weston Price, *Nutrition and Physical Degeneration* (La Mesa, California: Price-Pottenger Nutrition Foundation, 1954).
3. Schmid, op. cit.
4. Donald O. Rudin, M.D., and Clara Felix, *The Omega-3 Phenomenon* (New York: Rawson Associates, 1987).
5. Claudio Galli, and Artemis P. Simopoulos, *Dietary Omega-3 and Omega-6 Fatty Acids: Biological Effects and Nutritional Essentiality* (New York and London: Plenum Press, 1988).
6. Artemis P. Simopoulos, "Omega-3 Fatty Acids in Health and Disease and in Growth and Development," *American Journal of Clinical Nutrition,* 54 (1991): 438–63.

CHAPTER 15

# Cosmetics, Massage Oils, and Essential Oils

## Cosmetics and Rendered Fats

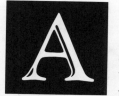 shocking story I have uncovered in researching this book is the tale of rendered oils. Rendering plants are large factories where tankloads of cooking oils and grease, collected from restaurants and fast-food establishments, are brought and processed. To these oils are added the fat from livestock and poultry deemed unfit for human consumption—animals that had cancer and other diseases. And last but not least, there are the deceased pets gathered from veterinary clinics, road kills, and the tens of thousands of dead cats and dogs, the euthanized strays from animal shelters.

The dead animals are dumped into huge cooking pots and roasted until the fat bubbles up from their bodies. Then the fat is collected, processed, and mixed with the processed oils from restaurants. Finally, these oils are sold to some of the leading cosmetic companies. These oils are a main ingredient in many of the most glamorous cosmetics, lipsticks, skin lotions, and soaps on the market. Not a pretty picture when you consider that most things put on your skin are absorbed into the body.

Some one billion pounds per week of animal by-products are processed into oils for use in various industries as follows: 42 percent in livestock feed; 25 percent in consumer and industrial products such as cosmetics, paint and rubber; 15 percent in soap; 10 percent in pet food; and 8 percent in other unspecified products. Indeed, many cat and dog foods contain meat and fat by-products from their dead cousins.

## Massage Oils

Massage therapy is one of the most ancient forms of healing known to man. Many renowned healers have recommended massage with therapeutic oils as one of the most important healing therapies available for a wide assortment of illnesses. Edgar Cayce frequently prescribed massage with healing oils—with great success—for arthritis, exhaustion, balancing the nervous system, muscular disorders, and many other conditions. He also observed that a good massage has the restorative effect of four hours' sleep. Yet, while many people are receiving what they consider to be a healing, therapeutic massage, they are, in fact, having poisonous substances rubbed into them.

Just to give you an idea of the situation, let's take a look at the almond oil used in massage therapy. Almond oil is considered to be one of the highest quality massage oils available, and yet all almond massage oil made in North America (except that made by Omega Nutrition in Ferndale, Washington) is not only processed, cooked, refined, deodorized, oxidized, and free radicalized, it is also made from nonorganic almonds that are full of pesticide residues and have a low mineral profile. To top it all off, it is not even made from food grade almonds, but rather from bug- and worm-infested chunks and pieces—discards or inedibles. Think about it for a minute. Do you want to have poisonous trans fatty acids, free radicals, pesticides, and extracts of worm carcasses rubbed onto your body?

Nearly all skin lotions today are also made from these toxic, nutrient-deficient refined oils. Even the most expensive skin-care products with the most sophisticated, glamorous advertising, including the so-called natural or healthy skin lotions, are made from refined oils.

The good news is that four companies—Omega Nutrition, Organic Marketing (formed by Fred Rohe), Advanced Nutritional Sciences, and Natures Symphony, one of the oldest aromatherapy businesses in the U.S.—have all brought out massage oils and skin-care products made entirely from organic, fresh-pressed Omega Nutrition oils. Sunrider International, Arbonne, and a few other companies make excellent animal-free cosmetics.

## Essential Oils

The essential oils that Natures Symphony and Organic Marketing use in their formulas are all imported directly from the south of France, the heart of the essential oil industry. The essential oils are gathered there from all over the world, using the best source for each oil. These oils are guaranteed to be produced from wild or organically grown flowers or herbs, and processed through simple, low-temperature distillation methods without the use of chemical solvents. These essential oils have remarkable properties for healing the physical, emotional, mental, and psychic levels of our being.

Geri Whidden, the founder and manager of Natures Symphony, gives the following description of essential oil processing methods:

> Most of the vegetable oils and essential oils on the market are of a "commercial" grade. To be of the highest quality, essential oils should be prepared from wild or organically grown plants. When pesticides are used on plants, they become concentrated in the oils.
>
> Where the plant is grown will alter its chemical constituents. For instance, if a plant is growing wild, high in the mountains and its sister is growing near the sea, their chemical

constituents and, therefore, healing properties will be very different. When the plant is picked will also greatly affect quality. Roses must be picked between dawn and noon, or half of their essential oil will have moved out of the flower. How soon the distillation is made after picking the flower is also important. For some plants like lavender, the distilling equipment is rolled out into the fields to capture the best quality. On the other hand, some flowers, such as orange blossoms, will produce more and better oil if given some time to dry first.

The length of distillation can also affect quality. The commercial oils are often "hurried" along, while better producers slowly distill the plant to capture a "whole symphony" of fragrance and energy.

Essential oils must be protected from temperature changes and light which influence their quality. Furthermore, many of the commercial oils are diluted with an oil solvent, or they can be altered or diluted with similar but cheaper oils. For instance, lemon verbena, which is expensive, is often diluted with lemon grass, which has a similar fragrance but is much cheaper.

Another common practice is the construction of an oil from the isolation of chemical constituents from other plants. These oils can be called "natural" because they come from natural sources. However, these oils do not have the healing effect of the oil which comes from the "real" whole, individual plant, and they should not be used for treatment.

Still other oils are synthetic and should definitely not be used for therapeutic purposes.

All of these products have their place and use, but only the finest quality should be used in healing work. These oils should be bought only from someone you trust who guarantees their quality. Unfortunately, there is a lot of adulteration in the essential oil business.

All of the oils made by Omega Nutrition, Omega / Arrowhead, Flora, and Seymour Organic Foods can be used for massage. Flax seed oil should be used in moderation, though, as an excessive amount can disturb the Omega-6 / Omega-3 ratio. The best oils for massage are almond, hazelnut, sesame, canola, and olive, or a combination of oils using the right proportion of flax seed with other oils. The Essential Balance blend is also a good formula to use. A small amount of high quality essential oil (fifteen to twenty-five drops to two ounces of base oil) can be added for its special healing properties.

Following is a list of some of the best essential oils to add to your oils for healing massages:

**Cypress** is an excellent choice for a massage before bed because of its calming, sedative effect. It soothes muscular cramps and the swelling associated with rheumatism. It helps improve circulation and eliminates fluid retention and cellulite. Its antispasmodic action quiets coughs, diarrhea, and menstrual cramps. Cypress strengthens broken capillaries and varicose veins. Do not massage veins. Apply oil by gently gliding over and around them. (Caution: avoid if you have high blood pressure.)

**Eucalyptus** helps to rebalance and improve energy and helps to prevent drowsiness. It is especially cleansing for people who work with chemicals. For the respiratory system, it fights and prevents colds, eases tight, dry coughs, flu, fever, and headaches. Its anti-inflammatory properties help relieve muscular aches, pains, rheumatism, and arthritis. It has an affinity for the urino-genital tract, and strengthens kidneys.

**Geranium** is another versatile tonic oil, uplifting to the spirits. It alleviates anxiety and depression and stimulates and regulates hormone production. Therefore, it is recommended for PMS, menopausal symptoms, fluid retention, cellulite (with rosemary), and to help eliminate toxins from the system. It is cleansing to liver and kidneys, and helps poor elimination.

**Lavender** is the most versatile oil—balancing and normalizing to body, mind, and spirit. It is recommended for general debility, stress, anxiety, depression, headaches, colds, and flu. It assists the lymphatic system in the elimination of toxins. It strengthens the function of the stomach, heart, gall bladder, lungs, and the body's defense system. It soothes muscular aches and sprains (and is especially good combined with rosemary and juniper).

**Rosemary** is a stimulating oil, especially recommended for fatigue, headaches, general aches and pains, and sprains. It helps improve circulation and lymphatic congestion, fluid retention, cellulite, and varicose veins. Its antispasmodic effect helps relieve colds, cough, and flu. It stimulates the liver, helps indigestion, flatulence, and constipation. It benefits the heart, gall bladder, and brain, and strengthens the central nervous system. It helps regulate the menstrual cycle. (Caution: avoid during the first month of pregnancy.)

**Sandalwood** is considered a sacred fragrance in the Orient. It is a calming, uplifting oil especially helpful for anxiety, depression, and fatigue. A hormone regulator, it is also useful for respiratory and urinary infections. It is a good massage oil for dry, mature, wrinkled skin.

You can buy massage oils and skin care lotions ready-made by Omega Nutrition, Organic Marketing, Sunrider International, Advanced Nutritional Sciences, or Natures Symphony. (For ordering information, see *Sources of Products* in the back of this book.)

ॐ

CHAPTER 16

# Summary

I t is not the intention of this book to propose that nutritional deficiencies are the sole cause of modern diseases. Obviously, there are other factors that play essential parts in health and illness. Meaningful work, exercise, self-love, honesty, inner peace, and living one's life in a conscious, responsible way all contribute to maintaining good health. Deficiencies of essential nutrients, pathogenic organisms, environmental poisons, poisons in foods, and undue social stresses are all negative forces that can undermine our health. This book explores just one aspect of the entire picture.

Many researchers have found that today's diets are seriously deficient in certain vital nutrients. Nutritional deficiencies of vitamins, minerals, enzymes, proteins, and fatty acids are a major cause of most current illnesses.

A primary concern in any nutritional program is the inclusion of adequate amounts of the Omega-3 and Omega-6 essential fatty acids. Indispensable for good health, we must obtain both from what we eat.

Studies have found that the main nutrient most of us are deficient in is the Omega-3 fatty acid. An inadequate intake of this nutrient has been established as a main cause of most modern diseases. Today, because of food processing, the average diet contains only one-sixth the amount needed and one-sixth the amount the average diet contained in 1820. (And in many diets, one-twentieth to one-hundredth the amount needed.)[1]

Just as an excess of cholesterol with an insufficient amount of Omega-3s can cause an imbalance, so too can an excess amount of Omega-3 fatty acids. Some Eskimos develop a condition in which their cellular membranes become so permeable that the fluid leaks out, and the slightest abrasion will cause swelling and leakage of fluid into tissues.

There are only two main sources of Omega-3 fats: cold water fish oils and organic flax seed oil. Flax seed oil is the richer source of Omega-3 fats: it requires less processing, tastes better, contains no toxic substances or cholesterol, is more stable, and is less expensive.

The correct dosage of flax seed oil is one to two tablespoons daily as a maintenance dose. This is a general amount. One should consider factors like age, size, and weight of the individual, dietary history, present diet, quantity of cholesterol normally consumed, quantity of cold-water fish normally consumed.

The Omega-6 fatty acids are also of critical importance in maintaining good health. Most of us eat ample (if not excessive) amounts of Omega-6 fatty acids, but insufficient amounts of Omega-3s. Omega-6s must be taken with an adequate amount of Omega-3s or they can have a deleterious effect on health. An acceptable ratio among researchers is about four to six parts Omega-6 to one part Omega-3 in the diet.[2,3] Although some historical diets point more to a one-to-one ratio.[4]

The Omega-9 fatty acid, mostly found in olive, hazelnut, sesame, and almond oil has long been valued for its beneficial effect on liver and gall bladder function. Its use is recommended to provide a good source of energy to the body and to help prevent heart disease.

GLA—gamma linolenic acid—supplies the body with the raw material to build certain prostaglandins. Borage seed oil is nature's highest source of gamma linolenic acid, more than twice as high as evening primrose oil. Sometimes, the best use of GLA is in small amounts for a short duration of time (one to three months), with plenty of supportive Omega-3s. Often, the body will regain its ability to produce GLA directly from the Omega-6 fatty acids. However, some people may need GLA on a long-term basis because of genetic malfunction, viral illness, or damage to their normal bodily processes. One should always take adequate Omega-3 fats with GLA or one may develop the problems caused by an Omega-3 deficiency.

To insure that we do not burden our bodies with toxic substances and that we receive adequate intake of our essential fatty acids, we should use only high quality oils with extra flax seed oil and/or include regular amounts of cold water fatty fish in our diets.

The elimination of any sources of oils containing poison-ous trans fatty acids, hydrogenated fats, free radicals, rancid fats, pesticide and herbicide residues, solvent residues, and other toxic substances is also necessary. This includes all commercial vege-table oils and almost all health-food store oils.

Of all the foods that we consume, none is as severely processed and converted into poisonous substances as are the fats and oils. Use of high temperatures and chemical solvents, as well as exposure to light and oxygen in the processing methods of nearly all oils produced today, destroys much of the Omega-3 and -6 essential fatty acids, and creates rancidity, poisonous trans fatty acids, and many other toxic compounds.[5,6,7]

Many companies today are producing poisonous oils by cheap processing methods, misleading the public into thinking they are cold-pressed by putting the oils into pretty bottles and selling them to the health food stores.

High quality oils need to be expeller-pressed at temper-atures below 118 degrees F instead of solvent-extracted. They should not be subjected to high heat temperatures, to deodor-izing, bleaching, alkali refining, or winterizing processes. They need to be produced by light and oxygen-excluding methods, bottled in containers that prevent further exposure to light (caus-ing rancidity), and, where possible, they should be produced from third-party, certified organically grown seed.[8]

At this time, I have found only two companies producing oils that meet these standards of quality: Flora Oils (Canada and U.S.) and Omega Nutrition (Canada and U.S.)/ Omega Nutri-tion/Arrowhead Mills (U.S.). Omega Nutrition/Arrowhead

Mills has the added advantage of oils bottled in completely light-excluding containers. Omega Nutrition and its distributors, Arrowhead Mills and other companies, are the only companies that have independent third-party certification (FVO and OCIA), because they use only organically grown nuts and seeds. These oils are available for purchase or can be ordered from your local health food or grocery store.

Several decades ago, Rachel Carson wrote a prophetic book entitled *Silent Spring*. Having ignored her (and other seers), we are now experiencing the tremendous damage to our crops and health that widespread use of pesticides, herbicides, fungicides, and synthetic fertilizers have brought upon us.

Why does mankind so often ignore the obvious warnings and the help offered by its prophets and visionaries? What will it take for people to understand that we must show a love and regard for the earth and the nourishment of our children, or we will pay for it in the future when they grow up with widespread disease, drug addiction, and violence?

It is critical that we care for and nourish the vital ecology of our spirits, our own bodies, our homes, our social system, and the earth itself by using wholesome processes in the growing and preparing of foodstuffs.

ぞ♪

This has been a tremendous journey for me, learning about the richness of nature in her many oils and the roles they play in maintaining good health and helping to cure disease. It has been very heartwarming to find out about companies with so much honor and conviction, who have worked hard and fought innumerable battles in their determination to give the public a real choice by providing exceptional products.

ﻫ

1. Donald O. Rudin, M.D., and Clara Felix, *The Omega-3 Phenomenon* (New York: Rawson Associates, 1987).
2. Claudio Galli, and Artemis P. Simopoulos, *Dietary Omega-3 and Omega-6 Fatty Acids: Effects and Nutritional Essentiality* (New York and London: Plenum Press, 1988).
3. Rudin, op. cit.
4. Artemis P. Simopoulos, "Omega-3 Fatty Acids in Health and Disease and in Growth and Development," *American Journal of Clinical Nutrition,* 54 (1991): 438–63.
5. Mensink and Katan, "Trans Fatty Acids and Lipoprotein Levels," *New England Journal of Medicine,* Vol. 323, No. 7 (August 16, 1990).
6. Daniel Swern, Editor, *Bailey's Industrial Oil and Fat Products* (New York: John Wiley and Sons, 1979).
7. Ann Louise Gittleman, M.A., *Beyond Pritikin* (New York: Bantam, 1989).
8. Theodore Wood Carlat, *Organically Grown Food* (California: Wood Publishing, 1990).

# Sources of Products

The following companies are the only ones that have FVO-, OCIA-certified organic oils, packaged in light-insulated containers:

## Omega Nutrition

United States:

1720 La Bounty Road
Ferndale, WA 98248
(206) 384-1238
FAX (206) 384-0700

Distribution: United States, Canada, and International. Produces and distributes a full line of FVO-, OCIA-certified organic fresh-pressed vegetable oils and ground flax seed meal (Nutri-Flax) in completely light-insulated containers.

Canada:

8392 Prince Edward Street
Vancouver, B.C.
Canada V53R9
(604) 322-8862
(800) 661-3529
FAX (604) 327-2932

## Omega Nutrition
## Professional Products Division

United States:

720 East Washington Street, Suite 105
Sequim, WA 98382-9917
(800) 745-8580

Distributes Essential Balance, other essential fatty acid formulas, and quality nutritional products for the professional market in the United States.

The following distribute Omega products:

## Advanced Nutritional Sciences

carries all mentioned oils, formulas, and books

Box 6712
Malibu, CA 90265
(800) 484-9828, ext. 4242

## Arrowhead Mills, Inc.

United States:

P.O. Box 2059
Hereford, TX 79045
(806) 364-0730
(800) 858-4308
FAX (806) 364-8242

Distribution: United States and International. Distributes the full line of Omega Nutrition FVO-, OCIA- certified organic fresh-pressed vegetable oils and Nutri-Flax, packaged in completely light-insulated containers. Also the largest producer and distributor of certified organic foods (grains, flours, beans, cereals, peanut butter, etc.) in North America.

## Natures Symphony

United States:

48 NE First Avenue
Boca Raton, FL 33432
(407) 393-0065
FAX (407) 482-5362

Distribution: United States, Canada, and International. Distributes massage and body oils made from fresh-pressed FVO-, OCIA-certified organically grown Omega Nutrition vegetable oils, mixed with essential oils extracted from wild or organically grown sources. Also distributes an exceptional line of organically grown or wild-gathered, properly extracted essential oils.

## Organic Marketing

United States:

15810 Shawnee Circle
Middletown, CA 95461
(707) 928-4098
FAX (707) 928-4740

Produces and distributes a quality line of skin-care products, incorporating OmegaFlo oils, French essential oils, and Chinese herbal extracts.

The following are not FVO-, OCIA-certified but claim to use third-party certified organic seeds and produce fresh-pressed oils in amber glass containers:

**Flora, Inc.**

United States:

Box 590
Lynden, WA 98264
(206) 354-2110
(800) 446-2110
FAX (206) 354-4110

Distribution: United States, Canada, and International. Produces and distributes a full line of fresh-pressed vegetable oils packaged in amber glass containers. Also distributes a full line of exceptional supplements, herb teas, and other nutritional formulas.

Canada:

7400 Fraser Park Drive
Burnaby, B. C.
Canada V5J5B9
(604) 438-4394
FAX (604) 438-4394
(800) 663-0617 Western Canada
(800) 387-7541 Ontario
(800) 363-9542 Quebec

**Ethical Nutrients-Metagenics**

United States:

23180 Del Lago
Laguna Hills, CA 92653
(800) 692-9400

Produces and distributes a full line of nutritional formulas, including the Opti, UltraClear, UltraBalance and UltraMeal formulas.

**Lifephase, Inc.**

520 Washington Blvd. Suite 455
Marina Del Rey, CA 90292
(310) 301-0033
FAX (310) 301-9697

**Source Naturals**

23 Janis Way
Scotts Valley, CA 95066
(408) 438–6851
(800) 776–7701

**Sunrider International**

United States:

3111 Lomita Boulevard
Torrance, CA 90505
(213) 534–4786
FAX (213) 530–4826

Produces and distributes a full line of exceptional quality Chinese herbal formulas.

For more information contact
**Price Pottenger Nutrition Foundation**
PO Box 2614
La Mesa, CA 92044–2614
*send legal-sized stamped, self-addressed envelope
(52 cents postage) and $6 for a list of physicians
who include nutrition in their therapeutic approach*

# Glossary

**Alpha-linolenic Acid:** The Omega-3 essential fatty acid. It cannot be made by the human body and must be obtained in the diet to maintain good health. It is found in marine plants and animals and cold-climate plants: nuts, seeds, and cereals. Flax seed oil is the highest source of alpha-linolenic acid.

**Arachidonic Acid:** An unsaturated fat made from the Omega-6 fat by enzymes in the body. Also found in meat. The prostaglandin 2 series is derived from arachidonic acid.

**Arteriosclerosis:** Hardening of the arteries.

**Atherosclerosis:** Deposits of cholesterol and fat containing plaque on the inside walls of the arteries.

**Beriberi:** A disease caused by an insufficient amount of Vitamin B1 (thiamine) in the diet.

**Beta Carotene (pro-vitamin A):** A precursor of vitamin A found in plant foods such as carrots, green leafy vegetables, and algae. More and more research is revealing its crucial role as an antioxidant that prevents free radical damage to cholesterol and helps to prevent and cure cancer. Normally present in high amounts in most vegetable oils, it is removed in the refining process. Fresh-pressed oils preserve the beta carotene.

**Bursitis:** Inflammation of the membranes of bursa, sacs made from tissues that protect tendons where they meet with friction at the joints.

**Carbohydrate:** Starches and sugars. Most starches are composed of complex carbo-hydrates, and most sugars are made from simple carbohydrates.

**Carcinogen:** Toxic substance that causes cancer.

**Carotene:** See Beta Carotene.

**Chelate:** An organic compound with several small groups of atoms that can bind a metal atom such as magnesium, iron, or zinc.

**Cholesterol:** A type of steroid fat found in many foods derived from animals that is also produced by the human body. Cholesterol is essential for the good health of the body, as it is the precursor for some hormones and a main component of our cellular membranes, nerves, and other vital body tissues. Excessive cholesterol is considered to be a partial cause of several diseases, including cardiovascular disease.

**Depression:** Extreme and long-lasting feelings of melancholy.

**Diabetes:** A disease characterized by the body's inability to adequately burn carbo-hydrates, either because of inadequate insulin or a lack of nutrients needed for proper metabolic function.

**Diverticulitis:** Inflammation of the colon, when pouches develop in the lining and become inflamed.

**Docosahexaenoic Acid (DHA):** An essential fatty acid of the Omega-3 family, essential for the normal development of the fetus and infants. It is found in human mother's milk and certain cold-water fish.

**Eczema:** Rough, red skin rashes developing in patches and linked to inadequate dietary nutrients, especially the Omega-3 fats. Also caused by the body's inability to properly metabolize fats.

**Enzyme:** A catalyst that accelerates chemical reactions.

**Essential Fatty Acid (EFA):** A fatty acid the body must obtain from foods, as it cannot produce it itself. The Omega-6 and Omega-3 fats are considered to be the only two fats that are essential.

**Estrogen:** A female steroid hormone that helps regulate a woman's menstrual cycle and fertility. Produced by the ovaries and adrenal glands.

**Free Radical:** A highly reactive chemical compound that can cause great tissue damage, and more and more, is being considered a main cause of some diseases, as well as a cause of the aging process. It is created by radiation, environmental toxins, heat and chemical processing of foods, and normal bodily metabolic functions.

**Gastritis:** Inflammation of the lining of the stomach.

**High Density Lipoprotein (HDL):** A substance made from fats and protein that transports fats in the blood away from the tissues. A high level of HDL is associated with a low risk for cardiovascular disease.

**Hormone:** A chemical compound produced by different glands that regulates many vital body functions. Examples are thyroxine, adrenalin, estrogen, and insulin.

**Hydrogenated Fat:** An unsaturated fat, usually a vegetable oil, that has been processed with high heat and hydrogen to harden it. Margarine and shortening are made from hydrogenated fats.

**Hypoglycemia:** Low blood sugar.

**Immune System:** An integrated system of many bodily defenses, including the nervous system, hormones, and cells protecting the body from disease.

**Irritable Bowel Syndrome:** Chronic inflammation, malfunction, pain, diarrhea, and/or constipation in the digestive tract, not caused by an identifiable organic disease. Often caused by long-standing nutritional deficiencies, poor diet, stress, disturbance of the normal beneficial bowel flora, and often having an underlying infection from Candida albicans, other yeasts, and/or parasites. Also called spastic colon.

**Linoleic Acid:** An essential unsaturated fatty acid from the Omega-6 family that cannot be produced by the body and must be supplied in the diet. Found in many vegetable oils.

**Linolenic Acid:** An essential unsaturated fatty acid from the Omega-3 family that cannot be produced by the body and must be supplied in the diet. Its main source is flax seed or flax seed oil, also walnuts, pumpkin seeds, salmon, tuna, sardines, rainbow trout, and other cold-water fish.

**Lipids:** Fats.

**Low Density Lipoprotein (LPA):** A type of lipid–protein molecule that deposits cholesterol in artery walls and tissues. A high level of LDL is considered dangerous.

**Malignant:** Usually referring to cancerous conditions that spread and are life-threatening.

**Metabolism:** The sum of all the body's biochemical processes involved in creating energy and body tissues from food.

**Monosaturated:** Fats with only one area of saturation, the main one being the Omega-9 fat (oleic acid), which is present in high amounts in olive, hazelnut, sesame, and almond oils.

**Omega:** The last letter of the Greek alphabet. Used to describe the last carbon atom in a chain.

**Omega-3:** The family of essential fatty acids made from molecules in which unsaturation begins three carbons in from the end carbon.

**Omega-6:** The family of essential fatty acids made from molecules in which unsaturation begins 6 carbons in from the end carbon.

**Omega-9 (Oleic Acid):** A nonessential fatty acid present in olive, hazelnut, sesame, and almond oils.

**Osteoporosis:** Loss of calcium from the bone causing reduced bone strength and increased possibility of fractures.

**Ovary:** The female endocrine glands located on either side of the mid- to lower belly. They produce the female hormones, estrogen and progesterone, which regulate a woman's fertility, menstrual cycles, and other functions.

**Pellagra:** A disease caused by a deficiency of niacin (vitamin B3). Its main symptoms are dermatitis (skin disorders), dementia (mental illness), depression, diarrhea, and fatigue.

**Placebo:** A substance that has no specific chemical effect, used as a control to test the viability of other medicines.

**Polyunsaturated Fatty Acid (PUFA):** An unsaturated fat with two or more areas of unsaturation.

**Premenstrual Tension Syndrome (PMS):** A combination of emotional and physical disorders immediately prior to menstruation.

**Prostaglandin:** A group of hormone-like substances derived from essential fatty acids that regulate many body functions.

**Psychosis:** A severe dysfunction of one's mental and emotional capacities, including a serious perceptual distortion of reality.

**Recommended Dietary Allowances (RDA):** The amounts of nutrients recommended by the Food and Nutrition Board of the National Academy of Sciences as the optimum needed to stay in good health.

**Saturated Fat:** A type of fat that is solid at room temperature. Present mainly in animal tissues, butter, coconut oil, and palm kernel oils. Also unsaturated vegetable oils converted into saturated fats like margarine and shortening by infusing with hydrogen gas at high temperatures.

**Schizophrenia:** A condition characterized by distorted perceptions, multiple personalities, and flattened emotional response.

**Scurvy:** A disease caused by a deficiency of vitamin C.

**Stroke:** A condition of impaired brain function caused by a blood clot or a hemorrhage of the vessels in the brain.

**Substrate:** A chemical compound that is acted upon by another (e.g., an enzyme) to convert it into another substance.

**Trans Fatty Acid:** A toxic fat implicated as a causative factor in heart disease, cancer, and other diseases, created by refining and hydrogenation processes. Refined oils may contain up to 25 percent trans fats while margarines and shortenings may have up to 50 percent trans fats.

**Unsaturated Fatty Acid:** A fatty acid with one or more double bonds between carbon atoms in its chain.

જ

# Bibliography

Alberts, Bruce, et al. *Molecular Biology of the Cell*. 2d Edition. New York: Garland Publishing, Inc., 1989.

Aldercreutz, H. "Does fiber-rich food containing animal lignan precursors protect against both colon and breast cancer? An extension of the 'fiber hypothesis.'" *Gastroenterol*, 86 (1984): 761-6.

Ballentine, Rudolph, M.D. "Butter vs. Oil." *East / West Journal*, February 1988.

Barnes, Broda O., M.D., and Lawrence Galton. *Hypothyroidism: The Unsuspected Illness*. New York: Harper & Row, 1976.

Bates, Charles, Ph.D. *Essential Fatty Acids and Immunity in Mental Health*. Washington: Life Sciences Press, 1987.

Behan, Peter O., Wilhelmina M.H. Behan, and D. Horrobin. "Effect of high doses of essential fatty acids on the postviral fatigue syndrome." *Acta Neurol Scand*, 82 (1990): 209-216.

Behan, Peter O. and Wilhelmina M.H. Behan, "Essential Fatty Acids in the Treatment of Postviral Fatigue Syndrome." *Omega-6 Fatty Acids, Pathophysiology and Roles in Clinical Medicine*. Alan R. Liss, Inc., 1990.

Bendit, E. "The Origin of Atherosclerosis." *Scientific American*, 236-2 (February 1977): 74-85.

Bjerve K.S., Thoereson. "Linseed oil and cod liver oil induce rapid growth in a seven-year-old girl with a N-3 fatty acid deficient." JPEN, *J. Parenter, Enteral Nutr.*, September / October, 12(5) (1988): 521-5.

Brisson, G.J. *Lipids in Human Nutrition*. Inglewood, NJ: Burgess, 1981.

Budwig, Dr. Johanna. *Das Fettsyndrom* (The Fat Syndrome). Freiburg, Germany: Hyperion Verlag, 1959.

Budwig, Dr. Johanna. *Der Tod des Tumors* (Death of the tumor). Freudenstadt, Germany: Budwig, 1977.

Budwig, Dr. Johanna. *Der Tod des Tumors* (Death of the tumor. vol. 2. Documentation). Band 2, Die Dokumentation, Freudenstadt, Germany: Budwig, 1977.

Budwig, Dr. Johanna. *Die elementare Funktion der Atmung in threr Beziehung zu autoxydablen Nahrungstoffen* (The basic function of cell respiration in its relationship to auto-oxidizable nutrients [essential fatty acids and sulphur-rich proteins]). Freiburg, Germany: Hyperion Verlag, 1953.

Budwig, Dr. Johanna. *Fette als wahre Hilfe* (Fats as real help). Freiburg, Germany: Hyperion Verlag, 1972.

Budwig, Dr. Johanna. *Fettfibel* (Fat notebook). Freiburg, Germany: Hyperion Verlag, 1979.

Budwig, Dr. Johanna. *Flax Oil as a True Aid Against Arthritis, Heart Infarction, Cancer and Other Diseases*. Vancouver, Canada: Apple Publishing, 1992.

Budwig, Dr. Johanna. *Fotoelemente des Lebens* (Light energy in life processes). Innsbruck, Austria: Resch Verlag, 1979.

Budwig, Dr. Johanna. *Kosmische Kraefte gegen Krebs* (Cosmic forces against cancer). Freiburg, Germany: Hyperion Verlag, 1966.

Budwig, Dr. Johanna. *Krebs ein Fett-Problem* (Cancer is a fat problem). Freiburg, Germany: Hyperion Verlag, 1956.

Budwig, Dr. Johanna. *Laserstrahlen gegen Krebs* (Laser rays against cancer). Freiburg, Germany: Hyperion Verlag, 1968.

Budwig, Dr. Johanna. *Oel-Eiweiss Kost* (Oil-protein combination). Freiburg, Germany: Hyperion Verlag, 1955.

Cameron, E. and Pauling, L. *Cancer and Vitamin C*. New York: Warner Books, 1979.

Cameron, Ewan, Director, Cancer Nutriprevention Project. Linus Pauling Institute of Science and Medicine. A study, June 10, 1987.

Carlat, Theodore Wood. *Organically Grown Food*. California: Wood Publishing, 1990.

Carlson, D.J., T. Supruchuck, and D.M. Wiles, "Photo-oxidation of Unsaturated Oils: Effects of Singlet Oxygen Quenchers." Division of Chemistry, Nat. Res. Conl. of Canada: *J.A.O.C.S.*, vol. 53 (October 1976).

Carson, Rachel. *Silent Spring*. New York: Fawcett Crest Books, 1962.

Chishti, Hakim, G.M., N.D. *The Traditional Healer*. Vermont: Healing Arts Press, 1988.

Consumer Reports. "Olive Oil." October 1991.

Crawford, Michael, and David Marsh, *The Driving Force*. London: Mandarin, 1991.

Douglass, William Campbell, M.D. *Eat Your Cholesterol: How to Live Off the Fat of the Land and Feel Great!* Atlanta: Second Opinion.

Epstein, S. *The Politics of Cancer*. San Francisco, CA: Sierra Club Books, 1978.

Erasmus, Udo. *Fats and Oils*. Canada: Alive, 1986.

Erasmus, Udo. *Fats That Heal, Fats That Kill*. Designing Health, 1988.

Faria, J.A.F., U. de Viscosa, and M.K. Mukai, "Use of a Gas Chromatographic Reactor to study Lipid Photo-Oxidation." Rutgers University, New Jersey: *J.A.O.C.S.*, vol. 60, no. 1 (1983).

Finnegan, John. *The Facts About Fats: A Consumer's Guide To Good Oils*. California: Elysian Arts, 1992.

Finnegan, John, and Kathy Cituk, *Natural Foods and Good Cooking*. California: Elysian Arts, 1989.

Finnegan, John, and Daphne Gray, *Recovery From Addiction, a Comprehensive Understanding of Substance Abuse—with Nutritional Therapies for Recovering Addicts and Co-dependents*. California: Celestial Arts, 1990.

Finnegan, John. *Regeneration of Health*. California: Elysian Arts, 1989.

Finnegan, John, and Kathy Cituk, *Weight Management: A Balanced Approach*. California: Elysian Arts, 1992.

Finnegan, John. *Yeast Disorders*. California: Elysian Arts, 1989.

Fischer, William L. *How to Fight Cancer and Win*. Canada: Alive, 1987.

Galeotti, T. et al. *Membranes in Tumor Growth*. New York: Elsevier Books, 1982.

Galland, Leo, M.D. *Superimmunity for Kids*. New York: Delta, 1988.

Galli, Claudio, and Artemis P. Simopoulos, *Dietary Omega-3 and Omega-6 Fatty Acids: Biological Effects and Nutritional Essentiality*. New York and London: Plenum Press, 1988.

Gennis, Robert B. *Biomembranes Molecular Structure and Function*. New York: Springer-Verlag, 1989.

Gittleman, Ann Louise. *Beyond Pritikin*. New York: Bantam, 1989.

Graham, Judy. *Evening Primrose Oil*. New York: Thorsons, 1984.

Gunstone, Harwood and Padly. *The Lipid Handbook*. London: Chapman and Hall, 1986.

Haas, Elson M., M.D. *Staying Healthy with Nutrition*. Berkeley, CA: Celestial Arts, 1992.

Haas, Elson M., M.D. *Staying Healthy with the Seasons*. Berkeley, CA: Celestial Arts, 1981.

Hamaker, John D. *The Survival of Civilization*. California: Hamaker-Weaver, 1982.

Hoffer, Abram, M.D., Ph.D. *Orthomolecular Medicine for Physicians*. Connecticut: Keats, 1989.

Holman, Ralph T., Susan Johnson, Paul Ogburn, "Deficiency of essential fatty acids and membrane fluidity during pregnancy and lactation." *Biochemistry*, Proc. Natl. Acad. Sci. USA, vol. 88 (June 1991): 4835-4839.

Horrobin, D.F. *Essential Fatty Acids: A Review*. from Horrobin, D.F., ed. *Clinical Uses of Essential Fatty Acids*. London: Eden Press, 1982.

Horrobin, D.F. "Post-Viral Fatigue Syndrome, Viral Infections in Atopic Eczema, and Essential Fatty Acids." *Medical Hypotheses*, issue #32 (1990).

Independent testing done by Cantest, Vancouver, B.C., showing no transmigration of hydrocarbons from black plastic containers used by Omega Nutrition.

Innis, Sheila M., and Harriet V. Kuhnlein, "Long-chain n-3 fatty acids in breast milk of Inuit women consuming traditional foods." *Early Human Development*. Elsevier Scientific Publishers Ireland Ltd., 18 (1988): 185-189.

*JAOCS*. vol. 65, no. 4 (April 1988).

*JNCI*. vol. 77, no. 5 (November 1986).

Jensen, Bernard, and Mark Anderson, *Empty Harvest*. New York: Avery, 1990.

Johnston, Ingeborg M., C.N., and James R. Johnston, Ph.D. *Flax Seed Oil And The Power of Omega-3*. Connecticut: Keats Publishing, 1990.

Kirschmann, John D. and Favon J. Dunne, *Nutrition Almanac*. New York: McGraw-Hill, 1984.

Kousmine, Catherine, Dr. *Sauvez Votre Corps!* S.A. Editions Robert Laffont, 1987.

Kwiterovich, Peter O., Jr., M.D. *Beyond Cholesterol*. Baltimore and London: The Johns Hopkins University Press, 1989.

*The Lancet.* "Is Vitamin B6 an Antithrombotic Agent?" 1 (1981): 1299–1300.

*The Lancet.* 2 (July–Dec. 1964): 975–979.

Langer, Stephen E., M.D. *Solved: The Riddle of Illness.* Connecticut: Keats, 1984.

Leibovitz, Brian, Ph.D. "Nutrition: At The Crossroads." *Journal of Optimal Nutrition,* 1 (1992): 1.

Levander, O.A., Al.L. Ager, V.C. Morris and R.G. May. "Protective effect of linseed oil against malaria vitamin E-deficient mice." *Flax. Inst. of the U.S. Proc.* 53 (1990): 16–19.

Levander, O.A., Al.L. Ager, V.C. Morris and R. G. May. "Protective effect of ground flax seed or ethyl linolenate in a vitamin E-deficient diet against murine malaria." *Nutr. Res.* 11 (1991): 941–48.

Levander, O.A., Al.L. Ager, V.C. Morris, R. Fontela and R. G. May. "Suppression of malaria by dietary oxidant stress." *Proc. 5th Int. Congress on Oxygen Radicals.* Kyoto, Japan, in press, 1992.

Liebman, Bonnie. "Baby Formula: Missing Key Fats?" *Nutrition Action Healthletter,* October 1990.

Liu, C. CF, et al. "Increase in plasma phasonalipid DHA and EFAs as a reflection of their intake and mode of administration." *Pediatr. Res.,* 22 (1987): 292–6.

Malhotra, Dr. *American Journal of Clinical Nutrition.* 20 (1967): 462–475.

Mead, J.F. and A.J. Fulco, *The Unsaturated and Polyunsaturated Fatty Acids in Health and Disease.* Springfield, IL: Charles C. Thomas, 1976.

Mendelsohn, R.D. *Confessions of a Medical Heretic.* New York: Warner Books, 1979.

Mensink and Katan. "Trans Fatty Acids and Lipoprotein Levels." *New England Journal of Medicine.* vol. 323, no. 7 (August 16, 1990).

Page, Melvin E., D.D.S., and H. Leon Abrams, Jr. *Your Body Is Your Best Doctor!* Connecticut: Keats, 1972.

Palangyo, K. et al. "An Open Study of Essential Fatty Acid Therapy (Efamol Marine) in Patients with AIDS." (available from Efamol).

Pfeiffer, Carl C., Ph.D., M.D. *Nutrition and Mental Illness.* Vermont: Healing Arts, 1987.

Pfeiffer, Carl C., Ph.D., M.D. *Zinc and Other Micronutrients.* Connecticut: Keats, 1978.

Phelps, Janice Keller, M.D., and Alan E. Nourse, M.D. *The Hidden Addiction and How to Get Free.* Massachusetts: Little, Brown & Co., 1986.

Pottenger, Elaine, and Robert Pottenger, Jr., eds. *Pottenger's Cats: A Study in Nutrition* (edited writings of Francis Pottenger). La Mesa, California: The Price-Pottenger Nutrition Foundation, 1983.

Prevention Magazine. *New Encyclopedia Of Common Diseases.* Pennsylvania: Rodale, 1984.

Prevention Magazine Editors. *The Complete Book of Vitamins.* Pennsylvania: Rodale, 1984.

Price, Weston. *Nutrition and Physical Degeneration*. La Mesa, California: Price-Pottenger Nutrition Foundation, 1954.

Raheja, Bihari S. *The Lancet*. November 14, 1987.

Rhinehart, J.F. and L. D. Greenberg. "Vitamin B[6] Deficiency in the Rhesus Monkey, with Particular Reference to the Occurrence of Atherosclerosis, Dental Caries and Hepatic Cirrhosis." *American Journal of Clinical Nutrition.*, 4 (1956): 318.

Robbins, John. *Diet for a New America*. New Hampshire: Stillpoint, 1987.

Rodale, J.I., and Staff. *The Complete Book of Minerals For Health*. Pennsylvania: Rodale.

Rona, Zoltan P., M.D. *The Joy of Health, A Doctor's Guide to Nutrition and Alternative Medicine*. Hounslow Press: Toronto, Canada, 1991.

Rudin, Donald O., M.D., and Clara Felix, *The Omega-3 Phenomenon*. New York: Rawson Associates, 1987.

Schauss, Alexander G. *Diet, Crime and Delinquency*. California: Parker House, 1981.

Schmid, Ronald. *Traditional Foods Are Your Best Medicine*. New York: Ballantine, 1987.

Serfontein, W.J., et al. "Plasma Pyridoxal-5-Phosphaste Level as Risk Index for Coronary Artery Disease." *Atherosclerosis*, 55 (1985): 357-61.

Simopoulos, Artemis, M.D. *Nutrition Today*. March / April 1988 & May / June 1988.

Simopoulos, Artemis P. "Omega-3 Fatty Acids in Health and Disease and in Growth and Development." *American Journal of Clinical Nutrition*, 54 (1991): 438-63.

Sinclair, H.M. *Essential Fatty Acids*. London, England: Butterworths, 1958.

Smith, Russell L., Ph.D. with Edward R. Pinckney, M.D. *The Cholesterol Conspiracy*. St. Louis, MO: Warren H. Green, Inc., 1991.

Stier, Bernard. *Secretes des Huiles de Premiere Pression A Froid*. Canada: 1990.

Stoff, Jesse A., M.D. and Charles R. Pellegrino, Ph.D. *Chronic Fatigue Syndrome*. New York: Random House, 1988.

Strandberg, T.E. et. al. *JAMA*, 266:1225-1229.

Swern, Daniel, ed. *Bailey's Industrial Oil and Fat Products*. New York: John Wiley and Sons, 1979.

Szent-Gyorgyi, A. *The Living State and Cancer*. New York: Marcel Dekker Inc., 1978.

Teeguarden, Ron. *Chinese Tonic Herbs*. New York: Japan Publication, 1984.

The Linus Pauling Institute of Science and Medicine, Palo Alto, California.

Thompson, L. and M. Serrino. "Lignans in Flax Seed and Breast and Colon Carcogensis." Department of Nutritional Sciences, University of Toronto, Ontario, Canada.

Tierra, Michael, CA., N.D. *Planetary Herbology*. New Mexico: Lotus Press, 1988.

Tierra, Michael, C.A., N.D. *The Way of Herbs*. New York: Pocket Books, 1983.

Treben, Maria. *Health From God's Garden*. Vermont: Healing Arts, 1988.

Treben, Maria. *Health Through God's Pharmacy.* Austria: Wilhelm Ennsthaler, Steyr, 1987.

Vincent, Peter, Engineering Research Assistant, Technologist/Physicist. Study done at T.R.I.U.M.F. at the University of British Columbia facilities, 1987.

Warner, K., Mounts, T.L. "Flavor and Oxidative Stability of Hydrogenated and Unhydrogenated Soybean Oils. Efficacy of Plastic Packaging." *Journal of American Oil Chemists Society,* vol. 61, N.R.R.C., Agr. Research Ser., USDA (March 1984).

Weissman, Joseph D., M.D. "The X Factor." *New Age Journal,* March/April 1988.

Werbach, Melvyn R., M.D. *Nutritional Influences on Illness.* California: Third Line Press, 1987.

Williams, Lowell L. et al. "Serum Fatty Acid Proportions Are Altered During the Year Following Acute Epstein-Barr Virus Infection." *Lipids,* vol. 23, no. 10, (1988).

Williams, R.J. *Nutrition against Disease.* New York: Bantam Books, 1971.

Wysong, Dr. Randy. *Lipid Nutrition.* Michigan: Inquiry Press, 1990.

Yamamoto, Y., E. Niki, R. Tanimura, Y. Kamiya. "Study of Oxidation by Chemiluminescence. IV. Detection of Levels of Lipid Hydroperoxides by Chemiluminescence." *Journal of American Oil Chemists Society,* vol. 62, Dept. Reac. Chem. Fac. Engr., U. of Tokyo, Japan (August 1985).

૨૦

# Index

# How This Book Came to Be

In researching the material for this book, I visited and examined the production facilities and processing methods of both Flora and Omega Nutrition in Ferndale, Washington, and Vancouver, Canada. I was graciously received and given a great deal of information and help from Bob Walberg, President of Omega Nutrition, and Thomas Greither, the owner of Flora. I also had extensive interviews and discussions with Robert Gaffney and Bill Vincent of Omega Nutrition and Seigfreid Gurshe, publisher of *Alive* magazine and former co-owner of Flora.

I flew to Germany and spent a most informative day in discussions with the charming and renowned Dr. Johanna Budwig. I next contacted the Kousmine Foundation and, while unable to visit the facilities and the Director, Dr. Kousmine, my colleague, Dr. Barbara Bieber, had extensive conversations with Dr. Kousmine's staff, asking them questions and gathering research on my behalf.

I next visited Biogarden, one of Germany's largest natural foods distributors, and spent a day with their director Rosie Reitschuster discussing oil production and the quality of oils in the marketplace. Later, I drove to Denmark and visited the organic, biodynamic farm of longtime environmental activist Jorgen Uhrskov. Jorgen is one of my oldest friends and a force for integrity and inspiration within the European environmental movement.

Returning to the U.S., I sought out many of the leaders in the natural foods movement. I spoke at great length with Fred Rohe, who has a wealth of knowledge from a lifetime of work in the organic and natural foods industry.

I also contacted one of the nation's most well known producers of health food oils, but they declined to discuss their oil processing methods with me and refused to allow me to visit their facilities.

I had several discussions with Udo Erasmus, author of *Fats and Oils;* with Betty Kannen at OCIA; Hugo Skoppik at FVO; Christine Beaman at Allergy Resources; Clem Perrault, who runs the largest organic farm in western Canada; Terry Cole, owner of Harmony Naturals, an organic food distributor in New Zealand and Australia; Charlotte Gerson, director of the renowned Gerson Clinic; Dr. Stephen Langer, author of *Solved: The Riddle Of Illness;* Mark Weideman, a manager at Premier Edible Oils; Mrs. Rudin, the wife of Dr. Rudin, who is the coauthor of the exemplary book, *The Omega-3 Phenomenon;* Dr. Michael Winther at Efamol Research; and finally, Dr. Dan Roehm, who manages a cardiology clinic in southern Florida where he has personally witnessed the recovery of many patients from heart disease, cancer, obesity, and other diseases through the application of sound nutrition and the judicious use of flax seed oil.

I have also seen firsthand the improvement and recovery from various diseases by many friends and clients who have implemented good living and dietary practices, proper use of oils, and herbal and nutritional supplements.

Finally, I spent thousands of hours studying the fats and oils literature, including some thirty books and over two hundred articles and scientific journals.

I hope this information will benefit many people. The harmful effects of refined oils and essential fatty acid deficiencies are a major causative factor in heart disease, cancer, immune system weakness and most modern diseases that have affected hundreds of millions of people all over the world.

The fats and oils story may well be the greatest scandal of greed, disinformation and ignorance in the entire history of food production.

These are strong statements, but I urge the reader to examine the information for yourself and see what conclusions you reach.

John Finnegan

# About the Author

John Finnegan was born in Greenwich Village and raised in Woodstock, N.Y., in the jungles of Latin America, and on the beaches and in the redwoods of northern California. He began writing his first book when he was nine years old—the story of his family's journey from New York to Lima, Peru. They were the first people to drive the length of Central America, often having to cut their own road through the jungle with machetes, shovels, and pickaxes.

At nineteen, he began to research the biochemical basis of physical and mental illness, which included studying with many of this century's leading medical pioneers. He studied life sciences and social sciences at San Francisco State University and the College of Marin, and continued his studies with Dr. John Christopher, Dr. Broda Barnes, Wendell Hoffman, Piro Caro, and other medical practitioners.

He is the author of nine books, including *Recovery From Addiction*, which he coauthored with Daphne Gray, published by Celestial Arts. He lectures and conducts seminars, giving presentations at the 1992 Los Angeles Whole Life Expo and at the 20th Annual Cancer Control Society Convention, and has worked in several holistic medical centers as a nutritional and environmental consultant.

*Other books you may find helpful from Celestial Arts:*

RECOVERY FROM ADDICTION by John Finnegan and Daphne Grey
Alternative herbal and nutritional therapies for a wide range of addictions, from cigarettes to sugar to caffeine to hard drugs. Includes first-person accounts of how these treatments have worked for a variety of specific problems.   $9.95 paper, 192 pages

STAYING HEALTHY WITH THE SEASONS by Elson Haas, M.D.
One of the most popular of the new health books, this is a blend of Eastern and Western medicines, nutrition, herbology, exercise, and preventive healthcare. $12.95 paper, 252 pages

STAYING HEALTHY WITH NUTRITION by Elson Haas, M.D.
The long-awaited examination of how what we eat determines our health and wellbeing. Truly a complete reference work, it details every aspect of nutrition, from drinking water to medicinal foods to the latest biochemical research. $24.95 paper, 1,168 pages

MENOPAUSE SELF-HELP BOOK by Susan M. Lark, M.D.
Nearly all of the symptoms of menopause can be prevented or relieved using a variety of dietary and other natural techniques—without the reliance on drugs and hormones so common in America today. Dr. Lark shows how any woman can ease this transition with proper diet, exercise, and stress reduction techniques. $16.95 paper, 224 pages

PMS SELF-HELP BOOK by Susan M. Lark, M.D.
PMS is not imaginary, and it can be treated without drugs. Dr. Lark gives specific, detailed treatments for relieving over 150 symptoms, complete with nutritional recipes and meal plans, yoga and acupressure exercises, and tips for reducing stress.   $16.95 paper, 240 pages

GENTLE YOGA by Lorna Bell, R.N. and Eudora Seyfer
This book is especially designed for people with arthritis, stroke damage, or multiple sclerosis, those in wheelchairs, or anyone who needs a gentle, practical way to improve their health through exercise. The book is spiralbound to stay open while you work and includes over 135 helpful illustrations.   $12.95 spiral, 144 pages

Available from your local bookstore, or order direct from the publisher. Please include $2.50 shipping and handling for the first book, and 50 cents for each additional book. California residents include local sales tax. Write for our free complete catalog of over 400 books, posters, and tapes.

Celestial Arts
Box 7123
Berkeley, Ca 94707

For VISA or MASTERCARD orders call (800) 841-BOOK.